Study Guide

Understanding Pharmacology

Essentials for Medication Safety, Third Edition

M. Linda Workman, PhD, RN, FAAN

Linda LaCharity, PhD, RN

Study Guide prepared by:

Lorraine Kelley, DNP, RN
Nursing Faculty
Department of Nursing
Fortis Institute
Pensacola, Florida

ELSEVIER

ELSEVIER

3251 Riverport Lane
Maryland Heights, MO 63043

STUDY GUIDE FOR UNDERSTANDING PHARMACOLOGY:
ESSENTIALS FOR MEDICATION SAFETY, THIRD EDITION

ISBN: 978-0-323-79351-3

Senior Content Strategist: Brandi Graham
Content Development Manager: Danielle Frazier
Senior Content Development Specialist: Rae L. Robertson

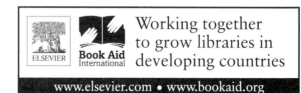

Printed in India
Last digit is the print number: 9 8 7 6 5 4 3 2 1

To the Student

This study guide was created to assist you in achieving the objectives of each chapter in the third edition of *Understanding Pharmacology: Essentials for Medication Safety,* and establishing a solid base of knowledge in pharmacology. Completing the exercises in each chapter in this guide will help to reinforce the material studied in the textbook and learned in class. Such reinforcement also helps students to be successful on licensure exams.

STUDY HINTS FOR ALL STUDENTS

Ask Questions!

There are no stupid questions. If you do not know something or are not sure, you need to find out. Other people may be wondering the same thing but may be too shy to ask. The answer could mean life or death to your patient. That is certainly more important than feeling embarrassed about asking a question.

Chapter Objectives

At the beginning of each chapter in the textbook are objectives that you should have mastered when you finish studying that chapter. Write these objectives in your notebook, leaving a blank space after each. Fill in the answers as you find them while reading the chapter. Review to make sure your answers are correct and complete. Use these answers when you study for tests. This should also be done for separate course objectives that your instructor has listed in your class syllabus.

Key Terms

At the beginning of each chapter in the textbook are key terms that you will encounter as you read the chapter. The key terms are in color the first time they appear significantly in the chapter. Phonetic pronunciations are provided for terms that students might find difficult to pronounce. The terms that were assigned simple phonetic pronunciations were selected because they are either (1) difficult medical, nursing, or scientific terms or (2) other words that may be difficult for students to pronounce. The goal is to help the student reader with limited proficiency in English to develop a greater command of the pronunciation of scientific and nonscientific English terminology. It is hoped that a more general competency in the understanding and use of medical and scientific language may result.

Key Points

Use the Key Points at the end of each chapter in the textbook to help with review for exams.

Reading Hints

When reading each chapter in the textbook, look at the subject headings to learn what each section is about. Read first for the general meaning. Then reread parts you did not understand. It may help to read those parts aloud. Carefully read the information given in each table and study each figure and its caption.

Concepts

While studying, put difficult concepts into your own words to see if you understand them. Check this understanding with another student or the instructor. Write these in your notebook.

Class Notes

When taking lecture notes in class, leave a large margin on the left side of each notebook page and write only on right-hand pages, leaving all left-hand pages blank. Look over your lecture notes soon after each class, while your memory is fresh. Fill in missing words, complete sentences and ideas, and underline key phrases, definitions, and concepts. At the top of each page, write the topic of that page. In the left margin, write the key word for that part of your notes. On the opposite left-hand page, write a summary or outline that combines material from both the textbook and the lecture. These can be your study notes for review.

Study Groups
Form a study group with some other students so you can help one another. Practice speaking and reading aloud. Ask questions about material you are not sure about. Work together to find answers.

References for Improving Study Skills
Good study skills are essential for achieving your goals in nursing. Time management, efficient use of study time, and a consistent approach to studying are all beneficial. There are various study methods for reading a textbook and for taking class notes.

ADDITIONAL STUDY HINTS FOR ENGLISH AS SECOND-LANGUAGE (ESL) STUDENTS

Vocabulary
If you find a nontechnical word you do not know (e.g., *drowsy*), try to guess its meaning from the sentence (e.g., *With electrolyte imbalance, the patient may feel fatigued and drowsy*). If you are not sure of the meaning, or if it seems particularly important, look it up in the dictionary.

Vocabulary Notebook
Keep a small alphabetized notebook or address book in your pocket or purse. Write down new nontechnical words you read or hear along with their meanings and pronunciations. Write each word under its initial letter so you can find it easily, as in a dictionary. For words you do not know or for words that have a different meaning in nursing, write down how they are used and sound. Look up their meanings in a dictionary or ask your instructor or first-language buddy. Then write the different meanings or usages that you have found in your book, including the nursing meaning. Continue to add new words as you discover them. For example:

primary
- of most importance; main: *the primary problem or disease*
- the first one; elementary: *primary school*

secondary
- of less importance; resulting from another problem or disease: *a secondary symptom*
- the second one: *secondary school (in the United States, high school)*

First Language Buddy
ESL students should find a first-language buddy – another student who is a native speaker of English and who is willing to answer questions about word meanings, pronunciations, and culture. Maybe your buddy would also like to learn about your language and culture. This could help in his or her learning experience as well.

Contents

Drug Therapy: Roles, Regulations, Actions, and Responses

chapter

1

LEARNING ACTIVITIES

Terminology Review

Match each definition with its corresponding term. (Answers may be used only once; not all options may be used.)

____ 1. A notice from the United States Food and Drug Administration that a drug may produce serious or even life-threatening effects in some people in addition to its beneficial effects

____ 2. The percentage of a drug dose that actually reaches the blood

____ 3. The science and study of drugs and their actions on living animals

____ 4. Drug action that is intended to kill a cell or an organism

____ 5. A substance that blocks the receptor site of a cell, preventing the naturally occurring substance from binding to the receptor

____ 6. A substance that activates the receptor site of a cell and mimics the actions of naturally occurring drugs

____ 7. The length of time a drug is present in the blood at or above the level needed to produce an effect or response

____ 8. Movement of a drug from the outside of the body to the inside through the skin or mucous membranes

____ 9. Movement of a drug from the outside of the body to the inside of the body by injection

____ 10. Movement of drugs from the outside of the body to the inside using the gastrointestinal tract

____ 11. The extent that a drug absorbed into the bloodstream spreads into the three body water compartments

____ 12. The removal of drugs from the body accomplished by certain body systems

____ 13. Movement of a drug from the outside of the body into the bloodstream

____ 14. The smallest amount of drug necessary in the blood or target tissue to result in a measurable intended action

____ 15. The lowest or minimal blood drug level

____ 16. Rapid inactivation or elimination of oral drugs as a result of liver metabolism.

____ 17. Refers to differences or variations in one person's specific gene or genes and how they affect the physiologic action of a drug

A. Agonist
B. Antagonist
C. Metabolism
D. Elimination
E. Pharmacogenetics
F. Distribution
G. First-pass loss
H. Black box warning
I. Peak
J. Trough
K. Minimum effective concentration
L. Duration of action
M. Cytotoxic
N. Enteral route
O. Parenteral route
P. Percutaneous route
Q. Pharmacodynamics
R. Pharmacology
S. Bioavailability
T. Absorption

Matching: Responses to Medications

Match the effect or response with its correct description. (Answers may be used only once.)

_____ 18. After taking an antibiotic, a patient developed an itchy rash.

_____ 19. After taking a sleeping pill, a patient was asleep for 6 hours.

_____ 20. A patient developed pseudomembranous colitis after taking antibiotics for 2 weeks.

_____ 21. A patient felt drowsy after taking an antihistamine.

_____ 22. A 72-year-old patient stayed awake all night after taking a sleeping pill. He reported feeling nervous.

_____ 23. A patient developed hemolytic anemia while taking a drug for malaria.

A. Paradoxical effect
B. Allergic response
C. Side effect
D. Adverse drug reaction
E. Idiosyncratic (personal) response
F. Therapeutic effect

Matching: Life Span Categories

Match the life span category to the correct issue or description. (Answers may be used more than once.)

_____ 24. Greater proportion of total body water

_____ 25. Need to avoid drugs that are teratogens

_____ 26. Reduced blood flow to the liver and other body areas

_____ 27. Reduced numbers of red blood cells and tissue oxygenation

_____ 28. May need a higher drug dose in terms of milligrams per kilogram of body weight

_____ 29. Placenta is not a perfect barrier

_____ 30. More likely to have a paradoxical reaction to a drug

_____ 31. Reduced rate of drug elimination

_____ 32. Problematic for drugs needed to manage chronic disorders

A. Pediatric consideration
B. Pregnancy/breastfeeding consideration
C. Older adult consideration

Identification: Drug Administration Routes

Specify below which drug delivery method and administration route goes with each description. (Drug Delivery options will be used only once; Administration Route options may be used more than once.)

Description	Drug Delivery	Administration Route
33. A tablet that is swallowed through the mouth		
34. A patch that is applied to the skin		
35. Injection into the fatty tissue below the skin		
36. Injection into the bloodstream through a vein		
37. Inhaled as a spray through the nose		
38. Injection into a muscle		
39. An injection into a body cavity		

Drug Delivery Options:
Intracavitary
Intravenous
Intramuscular
Nasal spray
Patch
Subcutaneous
Tablet

Administration Route Options:
Enteral
Parenteral
Percutaneous

Fill in the Blank

40. The _____, _____, _____, _____, _____, and _____ have the authority to write a drug prescription.

41. Disease of the _____ may affect drug metabolism.

42. A patient with severe kidney disease may have difficulty with drug _____.

43. The _____ of a drug is used to determine how much drug should be prescribed and how often it should be taken.

44. Newborn infants may have a slower rate of metabolism than an adult because the liver's _____ system is not yet fully active.

45. Infants have a(n) _____ proportion of total body water than adults.

MEDICATION SAFETY PRACTICE

Identify the correct drug pregnancy category (A, B, C, D, or X) for each description. (Each category will be used only once.)

____ 1. Drugs in this category have been shown to have an increased risk for birth defects or other problems in the fetus, but the drugs may be given if the benefits of treatment outweigh the risk.

____ 2. Drugs in this category are not to be given to women who are pregnant.

____ 3. Drugs in this category do not have an increased risk for birth defects or problems in the fetus.

____ 4. There have been no adequate studies in pregnant women, but animal studies have shown an increased risk for birth defects or other problems in the fetus.

____ 5. There have been no adequate studies in pregnant women, but animal studies have not shown an increased risk for birth defects or other problems in the fetus.

PRACTICE QUIZ

____ 1. A patient has been taking an opioid for severe pain for 3 days. This morning he says he is constipated. How is this effect described?
   A. Intended effect
   B. Side effect
   C. Adverse effect
   D. Paradoxical effect

2. Who is responsible for teaching patients about their drug therapy? *(Select all that apply.)*
   ____ A. Nurse
   ____ B. Unit secretary
   ____ C. Prescriber
   ____ D. Pharmacist
   ____ E. Nursing assistant

____ 3. Which describes the name of a drug that is created by the United States Adopted Name council, is relatively short and simple, and is not capitalized when written?
   A. Trade name
   B. Proprietary name
   C. Generic name
   D. Brand name

____ 4. The student is reviewing principles of pharmacology in preparation for a class, and is reading about the differences between intrinsic and extrinsic drugs. What is an example of an intrinsic drug?
   A. An oral drug taken to lower blood glucose levels
   B. Adrenalin secreted by the adrenal gland
   C. Intravenous opioids given to reduce pain
   D. Inhaled bronchodilators for asthma relief

____ 5. A drug is administered that will cause the same response as an intrinsic drug when it binds to the receptor of a cell. Which term best describes the action of the drug administered?
   A. Agonist
   B. Antagonist
   C. Cytotoxic
   D. Paradoxical

6. A patient is being monitored for an allergic or anaphylactic reaction after the first dose of an antibiotic. Which assessment finding(s) may indicate an allergic or anaphylactic reaction? *(Select all that apply.)*
   ____ A. Skin rash
   ____ B. Difficulty breathing
   ____ C. Hives on the skin
   ____ D. High blood pressure
   ____ E. Swelling of the mouth or throat
   ____ F. Bounding pulse

_____ 7. A dose of medication is to be administered sublingually. Which comment best explains the purpose of this route to a patient or family member?
   A. "The medication enters the bloodstream via the gastrointestinal tract."
   B. "The medication enters the bloodstream via the tissues under the skin."
   C. "The medication moves through muscles into the bloodstream."
   D. "The medication moves through oral membranes into the bloodstream."

_____ 8. A patient is receiving an intravenous injection of a pain medication. What is an advantage of the intravenous route?
   A. The drug goes straight to the liver for the first-pass effect.
   B. The drug enters the bloodstream quicker than the other routes.
   C. The intravenous route is safer than the oral route.
   D. Intravenous drugs are less expensive than oral drugs.

_____ 9. A patient who has one kidney is receiving morning medications. When assessing the patient for drug effects, the patient having only one kidney may result in which problem?
   A. Drugs may take longer to be eliminated.
   B. Drugs may take a shorter time to be eliminated.
   C. Drug metabolism may be increased.
   D. Drug metabolism may be decreased.

_____ 10. A patient has received a 500-mg dose of medication that has a half-life of 8 hours. How much drug is in the patient's bloodstream 16 hours from the time the medication was administered?
   A. 250 mg
   B. 125 mg
   C. 62.5 mg
   D. 31.25 mg

_____ 11. When administering drugs to infants and children, it is important to remember which principle of drug therapy?
   A. Most medication doses for infants are often higher in proportion than adult doses.
   B. Toddlers, preschool and school-age children, and adolescents usually have lower rates of metabolism than adults.
   C. An infant's kidneys will concentrate more water than an adult's kidneys.
   D. Water-soluble drugs are eliminated more rapidly in infants and young children than they are in adults.

_____ 12. An older adult is experiencing heart failure. Heart failure may cause what effect on the drugs that this patient is taking?
   A. The distribution of the drugs will be decreased.
   B. The metabolism of the drugs will be increased.
   C. The drugs will be absorbed slower.
   D. Heart failure will not have an effect on the drugs.

_____ 13. A health care instructor is teaching a class about drug therapy and pregnancy. During which stage of pregnancy is the risk of drug therapy causing birth defects highest?
   A. Weeks 1 and 2 of pregnancy
   B. Weeks 3 through 8 of pregnancy
   C. Weeks 9 through 20 of pregnancy
   D. The last 2 weeks of pregnancy

_____ 14. A patient asks about taking an herbal supplement to prevent colds. What is the best response?
   A. "Herbal supplements are safe, so you should be fine."
   B. "Just make sure you take this herbal product at least 2 hours after your morning medications."
   C. "Let's discuss this with your prescriber or pharmacist, as there could be interactions."
   D. "You should never take herbal products with your other medications."

15. The nurse's role in drug therapy includes which action(s)? *(Select all that apply.)*
     _____ A.   Select and order specific drugs.
     _____ B.   Dispense prescribed drugs.
     _____ C.   Administer prescribed drugs to the patient.
     _____ D.   Teach patients about ordered drugs.
     _____ E.   Know the purpose and adverse effects of drugs.

_____ 16. A patient asks why a certain medication is contraindicated while pregnant. What is the nurse's best response?
     A.   "Some medications may cause birth defects in the unborn."
     B.   "Your medical record shows you never took this medication."
     C.   "*Contraindication* means you have an allergy to the medication."
     D.   "An antidote is not available for this medication."

_____ 17. When reviewing an order for a high-alert drug, which is the nurse's best action before administering it?
     A.   Notify the provider to verify the order.
     B.   Double-check the dosage calculations.
     C.   Check the order with another licensed health care professional or pharmacist.
     D.   Administer a test dose initially.

Safely Preparing and Giving Drugs

LEARNING ACTIVITIES

Fill in the Blank: The Eight Rights of Safe Drug Administration

Each scenario reflects a problem with one of the eight rights of safe drug administration. Identify each "right" associated with the following descriptions.

1. The nurse was interrupted during morning medication rounds by an emergency. As a result, doses of morning medications were delayed by 3 hours. _____

2. The nurse reads the order for "Celebrex," then looks in the drug dispensing cabinet and pulls out "Celexa." _____

3. At the beginning of a new shift, the nurse sees that a medication that was due 2 hours ago was not signed off on the medication administration record. However, the patient insists that he did receive the medication. _____

4. During medication rounds, the nurse discovers that the patient is not wearing an identification wristband. _____

5. A patient is receiving an antibiotic, but actually has a viral infection only. _____

6. The prescriber gives a verbal order for "IV Lasix, now." _____

7. A patient says, "I don't know why I even bother taking this antidepressant. I'm still feeling depressed." _____

8. The nurse is reviewing orders written by the prescriber. One order states, "Give Tylenol, 650 mg, every 4 hours as needed for pain." _____

Matching: Administration Orders

Match the drug order with the correct drug order type. (Answers may be used only once.)

_____ 9. Levothyroxine, 50 mcg, by mouth daily

_____ 10. Valium, 5 mg, intravenous 30 minutes before the procedure

_____ 11. Morphine, 2 mg, intravenous, every 3 hours as needed for pain

_____ 12. Lasix, 40 mg, by mouth immediately

A. STAT
B. Standing
C. Single dose
D. PRN

Before or After?

For each action listed, mark whether the action is Before, After, or Both when giving a drug.

_____ 13.   Ask the patient about drug allergies.

_____ 14.   Check the residual amount of tube feeding remaining in the patient's stomach.

_____ 15.   Check the placement of the feeding tube.

_____ 16.   Flush the feeding tube with at least 50 mL of water.

_____ 17.   Ask the patient to gently blow his or her nose.

_____ 18.   Monitor the patient for therapeutic and adverse effects.

_____ 19.   Ask the patient to empty his or her bladder.

_____ 20.   Remove the old patch and any trace of previous doses.

_____ 21.   Check the patient's identification wristband.

_____ 22.   For rectally administered drugs, remind the patient to remain on his or her side for 20 minutes.

_____ 23.   Pull the earlobe up and out for children older than age 3 and adults.

_____ 24.   Wash your hands.

_____ 25.   Measure the liquid drug in a calibrated device.

_____ 26.   Document the drugs that were given.

_____ 27.   Select an appropriate needle for the injection.

Fill in the Blank: Parenteral Administration

Choose the most likely options for the information missing from the statements below by selecting from the lists provided. Each option will be used only once.

28. Intradermal drugs are injected _____1_____. The length of the needle is __2__ inch(es), and the gauge of the needle is __3__. The needle is inserted at a __4__-degree angle.

29. Subcutaneous drugs are injected _____1_____. The length of the needle is __2__ inch(es), and the gauge of the needle is __3__. The needle is inserted at a __4__-degree angle for most patients.

30. Intramuscular drugs are injected _____1_____. The length of the needle is __2__ inch(es), and the gauge of the needle is __3__. The needle is inserted at a __4__-degree angle.

Options for 1	Options for 2	Options for 3	Options for 4
Between the layers of skin	1-1.5	25-27	90
Deep into the muscle	3/8	20-22	10-15
Into the tissues between the skin and muscle	3/8	25	45

True or False: Drug Administration

State whether each statement is True or False. If the statement is False, explain why in the space provided.

_____ 31. Aspirate by pulling back on the plunger of the syringe after injecting a subcutaneous dose of heparin or insulin.

_____ 32. Intradermal drugs are given in the inner part of the forearm.

_____ 33. Remove the needle and discard the needle and syringe, without injecting the drug, if blood is seen in the syringe when aspirating during an intramuscular injection.

_____ 34. Place the sublingual tablet between the cheek and the molar teeth of the upper jaw.

_____ 35. When giving eardrops to a child younger than 3 years, pull the earlobe down and back.

_____ 36. Teach the patient not to swallow or chew a sublingual or buccal tablet while it is dissolving in the mouth.

_____ 37. A drug given by the intravenous route is injected directly into a vein.

_____ 38. The Z-track method for intramuscular (IM) injections is used for all IM injections.

_____ 39. After giving medications, reattach the nasogastric tube to suction.

Matching: Administration Routes

Match each intervention to its appropriate drug route using the options provided. (Answers may be used more than once, and not all options may be used.)

____ 40. Inject into the fatty tissues between the skin and the muscle layers.

____ 41. Use a 1- to 1.5-inch, 20- to 22-gauge needle for the injection.

____ 42. Be sure the patient can swallow.

____ 43. Use a 3/8-inch, 25-gauge needle, and 0.01 to 0.1 mL of fluid for the injection.

____ 44. Remove the old patch and clean the skin thoroughly.

____ 45. Have the patient lie down for 15 to 20 minutes after receiving the drug.

____ 46. Use the Z-track technique when injecting drugs that are irritating.

____ 47. Check the gastric residual before giving the medication.

____ 48. Place the tablet between the cheek and the molar teeth of the upper jaw.

____ 49. Stop the medication if fluid collects in the tissues.

____ 50. Do not give if the patient is experiencing diarrhea.

____ 51. Give the injection into the space between the epidermis and the dermis layers of the skin.

____ 52. Potential injection sites include the deltoid, vastus lateralis, and dorsogluteal areas.

____ 53. Use a 3/8-inch, 25- to 27-gauge needle with 0.5 to 1 mL of fluid for the injection.

____ 54. Wash hands.

A. Oral
B. Rectal
C. Intradermal
D. Subcutaneous
E. Intramuscular
F. Nasogastric tube
G. Intravenous
H. Buccal
I. Sublingual
J. Nasal
K. Vaginal
L. Topical/transdermal
M. All routes

MEDICATION SAFETY PRACTICE

For each statement or scenario, identify whether the action is Indicated or Contraindicated. If Contraindicated, rewrite the statement to make it an Indicated action.

_____ 1. After giving an injection, the cap is placed back on the needle before placing it into a sharps container.

_____ 2. The patient is in the bathroom when medications are given. The patient asks the health care worker to leave the medications on the bedside table, and the worker does as requested.

_____ 3. The nurse draws up an injection into a syringe, and then asks another health care worker to administer it because a different patient needs to be checked immediately.

_____ 4. The dorsogluteal injection site is selected for an intramuscular injection for an infant.

_____ 5. A drug error was made and immediately reported.

_____ 6. The patient states, "I can't swallow that capsule." The capsule is opened and given to the patient.

_____ 7. The person giving medications stays at the bedside until the drugs are swallowed.

_____ 8. The patient is assisted to the left modified left lateral recumbent position before giving a rectal suppository.

_____ 9. The deltoid site is selected to give a vaccination to a 16-year-old patient.

_____ 10. Before giving an intravenous infusion, the nurse removes all of the air from the tubing.

_____ 11. During medication administration, the patient states, "I don't recognize that pill. Are you sure it is right?" The order is checked before giving the medication.

PRACTICE QUIZ

1. A patient, who is new to the unit, is receiving medications. What should be done to ensure that the right patient is receiving the right drugs? (*Select all that apply.*)
   ____ A. Check the patient's name on the wristband.
   ____ B. Ask the patient to state his or her name and birthdate.
   ____ C. Check the patient's birthdate on the wristband.
   ____ D. Check the patient's identification number.
   ____ E. Check the patient's room number.

____ 2. A patient needs an oral dose of acetaminophen every 4 hours if the patient's oral temperature reaches 101.5° F (38.6° C) or greater. This is recognized as which type of order?
   A. PRN
   B. STAT
   C. Single
   D. Standing

____ 3. Prior to drug administration, a dosage calculation is performed. Which is the best action to prevent drug errors?
A. Use a calculator for the dosage calculation.
B. Perform the calculation twice.
C. Check the dosage calculation with a coworker.
D. Look up the dosage in a drug resource book.

____ 4. The nurse is administering morning medications and assess the patient first. The patient states, "Ever since I started that yellow pill, I've felt dizzy and nauseated." What should the nurse do next?
A. Assure the patient that this is normal.
B. Administer the drug.
C. Wait an hour before giving the drug.
D. Hold the drug and notify the prescriber.

____ 5. Medications will be administered through a nasogastric tube. When testing with an end-tidal CO_2 detector, the presence of CO_2 is noted. What should be the next action?
A. Administer the medications.
B. Flush the tubing with 50 mL of water.
C. Attach the tubing to suction.
D. Hold the medications.

____ 6. An intramuscular injection will be given to an adult patient. Upon checking the dosage, the volume of the injection is 3.2 mL. Which action is appropriate?
A. Give the entire amount in one injection.
B. Divide the dose and give two injections.
C. Use the Z-track method to administer the injection.
D. Hold the injection and notify the prescriber.

____ 7. A patient's family member is preparing to administer a topical cream to a patient's skin. Which action by the family member reflects a need for further teaching?
A. Performing handwashing and applying gloves before giving the medication
B. Cleaning the patient's skin before applying the medication
C. Shaving the patient's hair off the site before applying the medication
D. Applying a smooth, thin layer to the patient's skin

____ 8. A patient's wife is being taught how to administer eardrops to her husband. Which action by the wife indicates a need for further teaching?
A. Pulling the earlobe down and back to give the eardrops
B. Pulling the earlobe up and out to give the eardrops
C. Asking her husband to lie on his side for at least 5 minutes after giving the drops
D. Administering the drug without letting the ear dropper touch the ear

____ 9. Morning medications have been given to a patient with hypertension. Which immediate action is most appropriate at this time?
A. Checking the patient's blood pressure
B. Assessing the patient's pain level
C. Teaching the patient the purpose of the medication
D. Documenting the medication given

____ 10. Crushed oral medication will be given to a 3-year-old child. Which statement is appropriate?
A. "Here is some candy for you!"
B. "This medicine tastes really good!"
C. "Would you like to take it with apple juice or fruit punch?"
D. "Would you like me to mix this in a glass of orange juice?"

Mathematics Review and Introduction to Dosage Calculations

chapter

3

LEARNING ACTIVITIES

Terminology Review

Match each definition with its corresponding term. (Answers may be used only once; not all options may be used.)

_____ 1. The bottom number in a fraction

_____ 2. The top number in a fraction that is divided by the bottom number

_____ 3. The answer to a division problem

_____ 4. The expression of how a number is related to 100

_____ 5. The part of a whole number based on a system of units of 10

_____ 6. An equal mathematic relationship between two sets of numbers

_____ 7. A fraction that has a numerator that is lower than the denominator

_____ 8. A fraction that has a whole number with a fraction attached

_____ 9. A fraction that has been changed to the lowest common denominator

_____ 10. The number to be divided in a division problem

A. Proper fraction
B. Reduced fraction
C. Mixed-number fraction
D. Improper fraction
E. Dividend
F. Divisor
G. Decimal
H. Numerator
I. Denominator
J. Percent
K. Quotient
L. Proportion

Fill in the Blank

11. For the fractions listed below, identify the numerator and denominator, and specify whether the fraction is a proper or improper fraction.

    a. $\frac{5}{9}$

    Numerator: _____ Denominator: _____ Proper/Improper fraction? _____

    b. $\frac{9}{4}$

    Numerator: _____ Denominator: _____ Proper/Improper fraction? _____

c. $^{11}/_6$

Numerator: _____ Denominator: _____ Proper/Improper fraction? _____

d. $^2/_3$

Numerator: _____ Denominator: _____ Proper/Improper fraction? _____

12. For the decimal numbers listed below, identify the dividend, the divisor, and the quotient.

   a. $^{36.5}/_2$

   Dividend: _____ Divisor: _____ Quotient: _____

   b. $^{11.4}/_{5.9}$

   Dividend: _____ Divisor: _____ Quotient: _____

   c. $^{30.3}/_5$

   Dividend: _____ Divisor: _____ Quotient: _____

   d. $^{52.5}/_{4.6}$

   Dividend: _____ Divisor: _____ Quotient: _____

13. Change each number below to a fraction.

   a. 9 _____

   b. 552 _____

14. Change each mixed number fraction below to an improper fraction.

   a. $1\,^3/_4$ ——————————————————

   b. $5\,^1/_3$ ——————————————————

15. Reduce each fraction to its lowest terms.

   a. $^{75}/_{100}$ ——————————————————

   b. $^{99}/_{126}$ ——————————————————

   c. $^{53}/_{72}$ ——————————————————

   d. $^{12}/_{288}$ ——————————————————

16. Calculate the answer to each problem below. If the answer is an improper fraction, convert it to a mixed number fraction.

   a. $\frac{2}{3} + \frac{5}{3}$ ——————————————

   b. $\frac{1}{6} + \frac{2}{6} + \frac{3}{6} + \frac{5}{6}$ ————————————

   c. $\frac{2}{6} + \frac{3}{5} + \frac{1}{3}$ ——————————

   d. $\frac{6}{8} - \frac{4}{8}$ ——————————————

   e. $4\frac{3}{8} - \frac{12}{8}$ ————————————

   f. $7\frac{5}{8} - 2\frac{1}{5}$ ————————————

   g. $\frac{4}{8} \times \frac{1}{3}$ ——————————————

   h. $\frac{1}{8} \times 5\frac{1}{2}$ ——————————————

   i. $7\frac{1}{2} \times 4\frac{1}{5}$ ————————————

   j. $4 \div \frac{1}{2}$ ————————————————

   k. $\frac{7}{8} \div \frac{1}{3}$ ——————————————

   l. $7\frac{1}{4} \div \frac{3}{5}$ ——————————————

17. Calculate the product or quotient of each problem below.

   a. 0.125×100 ——————————————

   b. 11.4×5.9 ——————————————

   c. $\frac{1}{5} \times 3.8$ ——————————————

   d. $550 \div 0.2$ ——————————————

   e. $1.7 \div 1.7$ ——————————————

   f. $6.5 \div 0.35$ ——————————————

18. Change each fraction below to a decimal.

   a. $\frac{75}{100}$ ——————————————

   b. $\frac{1}{3}$ ——————————————

   c. $\frac{4}{5}$ ——————————————

19. Change each decimal below to a fraction.

    a. 0.25 —————————————————

    b. 0.88 —————————————————

    c. 0.46 —————————————————

20. Calculate the given percentages of each number below.

    a. 1% of 100 —————————————————

    b. 55% of 50 —————————————————

    c. 0.5% of 10 —————————————————

21. Express each problem below as a fractional proportion.

    a. If one batch of cookies yields 12 cookies, then 3 batches of cookies yields 36 cookies.

       —————————————————

    b. If 1 mL of filgrastim contains 300 mcg, then 2 mL contains 600 mcg.

       —————————————————

MEDICATION SAFETY PRACTICE

1. Identify which numbers are written correctly and which are written incorrectly. For the incorrect numbers, write them correctly in the space provided.

    a. 125.0   *Correct/Incorrect?* —————————————

    b. .1800   *Correct/Incorrect?* —————————————

    c. 0.67   *Correct/Incorrect?* —————————————

    d. 78.2400 *Correct/Incorrect?* —————————————

    e. 00.65   *Correct/Incorrect?* —————————————

2. If a dosage calculation results in the dosage being 1.5 scored tablets, how many tablets will be given? ————

3. The nurse is to administer 40 mg of promethazine IM before a procedure to prevent nausea. The medication is available in a vial of 50 mg/mL. How many mL will the nurse draw up in the syringe for this dose? ———— mL

4. The nurse is preparing to give a patient 0.5 mg of alprazolam PO. The medication is available in 1-mg tablets, which are scored. How many tablets will the patient receive? _____ tablet(s)

5. The provider has ordered 25 g of lactulose PO. The medication is a syrup that comes in unit dose packs of 10 g/15 mL. How many milliliters will the nurse administer? _____ mL

6. A medication order reads "Give 200 mg of allopurinol PO daily." The medication is available in 100-mg tablets. Use the proportion method to calculate how many tablets the patient would receive. _____ tablet(s)

7. What happens to a drug dose calculation if the decimal point is moved in error to the right?

_____

8. What happens to a drug dose calculation if the decimal point is moved in error to the left?

_____

PRACTICE QUIZ

_____ 1. In the formula $X = 45/90$, which element of the formula represents the numerator?
    A. X
    B. /
    C. 45
    D. 90

_____ 2. Of the fractions listed below, which represents an improper fraction?
    A. ½
    B. 1¾
    C. ⁷⁰⁄₃₅
    D. ²⁰⁄₁₀₀

_____ 3. Which fraction correctly represents the whole number 55?
    A. ⁵⁵⁄₁
    B. ¹⁄₅₅
    C. ⁵⁵⁄₁₀₀
    D. ⁵·⁵⁄₁

_____ 4. Which fraction correctly represents 6⅞?
    A. ¹³⁄₈
    B. ¹⁴⁄₇
    C. ⁵⁵⁄₈
    D. ⁷⁄₁₄

_____ 5. Which fraction is reduced to its lowest terms?
    A. ³⁄₉
    B. ⁵⁄₁₅
    C. ⁶⁄₇₂
    D. ⁴⁄₂₅

_____ 6. What is the lowest common denominator for this series of fractions: ⅝, ⅓, ½?
    A. 8
    B. 16
    C. 24
    D. 48

7. Calculate the answer to this problem: ⅝ − ⅗. Reduce the fraction to its lowest terms.

8. Calculate the answer to this problem: ⁴⁄₁₂ × ¹⁄₁₆. Reduce the fraction to its lowest terms.

9. Calculate the answer to this problem: ⅔ ÷ ⁵⁄₇. Reduce the fraction to its lowest terms.

_____ 10. In the equation $3.33 \div 2.25 = 1.48$, which element is the dividend?
    A. 3.33
    B. 2.25
    C. 1.48
    D. =

11. Calculate the answer to this problem: 11.4 × 12.6, rounded to tenths.

12. Calculate the answer to this problem: 7.17 ÷ 11.16, rounded to tenths.

_____ 13. Which number expresses the fraction ¾ as a decimal?
    A. 0.34
    B. 3.4
    C. .75
    D. 0.75

_____ 14. Which number expresses the decimal 6.3 as a fraction?
    A. ²⁄₁
    B. ⁶⁄₃
    C. 6 ³⁄₁₀
    D. ⁶³⁄₁

_____ 15. How much is 15% of 45?
    A. 0.675
    B. 6.75
    C. 67.5
    D. 675

16. The medication order reads "Nadolol, 180 mg, PO daily." The scored tablets are 120 mg/tablet. How many tablets will be given for this dose? _____ tablet(s)

17. The nurse is preparing to administer megestrol, 120 mg PO to a patient with chemotherapy-induced anorexia. The medication is available in unit-dose containers of 40 mg/mL. How much will the nurse administer? _____ mL

18. The medication order reads "Furosemide, 80 mg, PO now" for a patient with hypertension. The medication is available in scored 40-mg tablets. Using the proportion method, calculate how many tablets will be given for this dose. _____ tablet(s)

Medical Systems of Weights and Measures

LEARNING ACTIVITIES

Matching

Match each definition with its corresponding term. (Not all options may be used.)

_____ 1. A system of volume and weight measurements formerly used by medical professionals

_____ 2. Equal in amount or to have equal value

_____ 3. System of temperature measurement in which the freezing point of water is 32° above 0°

_____ 4. The basic metric unit for measurement of weight

_____ 5. The basic metric unit for measurement of length

_____ 6. System of temperature measurement in which the freezing point of water is 0°

A. Dimensional analysis
B. Equivalent
C. Celsius/centigrade
D. Gram
E. Liter
F. Apothecary
G. Fahrenheit
H. Meter

Fill in the Blank: Equivalents

Complete the following equivalents.

7. 1 pound = _____ ounces

8. _____ teaspoons = 1 tablespoon

9. 1 cup = _____ ounces

10. 1 gallon = _____ quarts

11. _____ feet = 1 yard

12. $32°\ F$ = _____ $° C$

13. 1 kilogram = _____ grams

14. 1 gram = _____ milligrams

15. 1 liter = _____ milliliters

16. 1 centimeter = _____ millimeters

17. _____ pounds = 1 kilogram

18. 1 teaspoon = _____ milliliter(s)

19. _____ drops = 1 milliliter

20. 15 milliliters = _____ tablespoon(s)

21. 1 fluid ounce = _____ milliliter(s)

Fill in the Blank: Prefixes

For each prefix list the correct unit of measure and its abbreviation.

22. "kilo"   Weight: _____   Length: _____

23. "micro"   Weight: _____

24. "deci"   Liquids: _____

25. "centi"   Length: _____

26. "milli"   Weight: _____   Liquids: _____   Length: _____

MEDICATION SAFETY PRACTICE

True or False

Mark each statement as True or False. If the statement is False, correct it to make it True.

_____ 1.   A liquid ounce is equal to a dry ounce.

_____ 2.   Patients may use teaspoons and tablespoons from tableware to measure liquid drugs.

_____ 3.   When measuring liquid drugs in a medicine cup, fill while holding the cup at eye level.

_____ 4.   A 1-milligram tablet of a drug is 1000 times stronger than a 1-microgram tablet of that same drug.

_____ 5.   A person's weight in kilograms is approximately double his or her weight in pounds.

_____ 6. The abbreviation "U" is acceptable for abbreviating "units" when dosing heparin.

_____ 7. Milliequivalents are used to measure electrolytes.

_____ 8. Insulin syringes may be interchanged with noninsulin syringes.

_____ 9. Normal human body temperature in Celsius/centigrade ranges between 36.1° and 37.8° C.

_____ 10. When giving liquid medication with a dropper, place the dropper into the side of the patient's mouth rather than in the middle where it can cause choking if it runs down the throat too quickly.

Conversions

Solve the following conversion problems, dosage problems, and drug calculations.

11. 100° F = _____ ° C

12. 39.5° C = _____ ° F

13. The nurse is to administer 2 tsp of cough syrup every 4 hours as needed to a patient with a cough. Convert 2 tsp to mL. _____ mL

14. 600 mL = _____ L

15. 2.5 L = _____ mL

16. 223 lbs = _____ kg

17. 79 kg = _____ lbs

18. 15 oz = _____ g

19. The nurse is preparing to administer a bolus injection of 8000 units of heparin to a patient with a blood clot. The vial of heparin contains 10,000 units/mL. How many milliliters will be drawn up into the syringe? _____ mL

PRACTICE QUIZ

____ 1. Which unit is the basic measure of weight in the metric system?
A. Dram
B. Gram
C. Meter
D. Liter

2. Which statements does the nurse realize are correct about metric measurements? *(Select all that apply.)*
____ A. A kilogram is 1000 times heavier than a gram.
____ B. A centimeter is 1/10 of a meter.
____ C. A milligram is 1000 times smaller than a gram.
____ D. A milliliter is 1/1000 of a liter.
____ E. A microgram is 1000 times heavier than a milligram.

____ 3. The nurse receives an order for a liquid medication that states to give "1 fluid ounce" per dose. The patient has a medication measuring device that is marked in tablespoons only. The nurse instructs the patient that the dose of 1 fluid ounce equals how many tablespoons?
A. ½
B. 1
C. 2
D. 3

4. Which units are appropriate measures for solids? *(Select all that apply.)*
____ A. Ounce
____ B. Teaspoon
____ C. Drop
____ D. Gram
____ E. Milliliter
____ F. Nanogram

____ 5. During a nursing admission assessment, the patient weighs 109.1 kg. The patient asks the nurse, "What does that mean in pounds?" Which answer is correct?
A. "You weigh 109.1 pounds."
B. "You weigh 218 pounds."
C. "You weigh 240 pounds."
D. "You weigh 272.8 pounds."

6. A patient reports constipation and the provider has given an order to give magnesium hydroxide, 1.5 ounces, at bedtime as needed. How many mL will be given to the patient? _____ mL

7. As part of a bowel preparation before a colonoscopy, a patient will need to take 15 doses of 200 mL of polyethylene glycol electrolyte solution every 10 minutes. After this prep is completed, how many liters of medication will the patient have consumed? _____ L

8. A patient will be receiving an intravenous dose of penicillin G potassium, 500,000 units per dose, every 6 hours. The medication is available in vials of 1 million units/50 mL. How many mL will the nurse draw up in the syringe to prepare an IV piggyback solution that contains 500,000 units of this medication? _____ mL

9. The nurse is preparing to administer a 10-mEq dose of oral potassium chloride liquid medication. The medication comes in unit dose packets of 20 mEq/15 mL. How many mL will the patient receive per dose? _____ mL

____ 10. Digoxin 250 micrograms PO is prescribed. The medication is available in scored tablets of 0.25 mg each. How many tablets should be given to the patient?
A. ¹⁄₁₀
B. ¹⁄₂₅
C. 1
D. 10

Dosage Calculation of Intravenous Solutions and Drugs

chapter

5

LEARNING ACTIVITIES

Matching: Terminology Review

Match each definition with its corresponding term. (Answers may be used only once; not all options may be used.)

_____ 1. How long (in minutes or hours) an IV infusion is ordered to run

_____ 2. Number of drops per minute needed to make an IV solution infuse in the prescribed amount of time

_____ 3. Number of drops needed to make 1 mL of IV fluid

_____ 4. Number of mL delivered in 1 hour of an IV infusion

_____ 5. Result of an infusion of IV fluids that occurs at a much faster rate than was ordered, causing harm to the patient

_____ 6. Leakage of irritating IV fluids into tissue surrounding the vein, resulting in tissue damage

_____ 7. Leakage of IV fluids into tissue surrounding the vein, resulting in tissue swelling

_____ 8. IV pump abbreviation for the volume of fluid that has already infused

_____ 9. Computer-based machine that pushes fluid into the vein by slow pressure

_____ 10. Device that uses gravity to control the flow of an IV

A. Controller
B. IV infusion pump
C. Fluid overload
D. Extravasation
E. Infiltration
F. Flow rate
G. Duration
H. Drop factor
I. Drip rate
J. VTBI
K. VI

Identification: IV Tubing Sets

For each tubing drop factor listed below, indicate whether the tubing that should be used is macrodrip or microdrip.

_____ 11. 10 drops/mL

_____ 12. 15 drops/mL

_____ 13. 20 drops/mL

_____ 14. 60 drops/mL

_____ 15. Used most often for children, older patients, and patients who cannot tolerate a fast infusion or a high volume of fluids

_____ 16. Used most often when fast infusion rates or larger quantities of fluids or drugs are needed

MEDICATION SAFETY PRACTICE

1. Which term is used to indicate how long in minutes or hours an infusion is to run?

2. The nurse is monitoring a patient who has an IV infusion that is due to be completed by 8 AM. It is now 9 AM and there is still 150 mL left in the IV bag. The nurse increases the infusion rate to make up for lost time. Which practices of safe medication administration has the nurse not performed?

3. The nurse has received a drug order from the provider that reads "Infuse 1000 mL of 0.9% normal saline IV over 12 hours." At which infusion rate in milliliters per hour would the nurse administer the IV fluids?

4. A patient is to receive D_5W with macrodrip tubing with a drop factor of 10 drops/mL. The order states: "Infuse D_5W 1000 mL over 10 hours." At which rate in drops per minute would the nurse administer the IV fluids?

5. The nurse is preparing to calculate the microdrip rate for an IV infusion order that states: "Infuse $D_5\frac{1}{2}NS$ at 50 mL/hour." How many drops/minute would the nurse administer the IV fluid?

6. The provider has prescribed IV fluids of 0.9% normal saline to infuse at 75 mL/hour for 24 hours. The nurse uses macrodrip tubing with a drop factor of 15 drops per milliliter. At which drip rate would the nurse administer the IV fluid?

PRACTICE QUIZ

____ 1. A patient is very restless while receiving IV fluids to treat dehydration. The IV catheter has slipped out of the vein and fluid is delivered to the surrounding tissues under the skin, causing swelling. Which term best describes this occurrence?
A. Infection
B. Fluid overload
C. Infiltration
D. Extravasation

____ 2. Which IV tubing set delivers the smallest drops?
A. 10 drops/mL
B. 15 drops/mL
C. 20 drops/mL
D. 60 drops/mL

3. Which components are required for an order for IV fluids? *(Select all that apply.)*
____ A. Type of fluid to be administered
____ B. Controller device
____ C. Volume to be administered
____ D. Duration of fluid administration
____ E. Rate of fluid administration

4. An IV order reads "Infuse 2000 mL of normal saline over 24 hours." With a tubing set drop factor of 10, what is the drip rate for this IV infusion? _____ gtts/min

____ 5. A patient received an intravenous solution that led to tissue damage. What is the term used to describe this?
A. Infiltration
B. Extravasation
C. Fluid overload
D. IV pump failure

6. Using the "15-second" rule, calculate the drip rate for an IV infusion of 150 mL/hour. The tubing has a drip factor of 20. _____ gtts/min

7. An IV is to infuse at 36 drops per minute. How many drops should be counted in 15 seconds? _____ gtts in 15 seconds

____ 8. A patient is to receive intravenous fluids at a rate of 100 mL/hr. When the IV pump is programmed, a rate of 150 mL/hr is set. What will most likely occur?
A. The computer will recognize the error and ignore the setting.
B. An insufficient amount of fluids will be infused.
C. The pump will alert the nurse to the error in the setting
D. The pump will infuse the fluid at the settings as programmed.

____ 9. The following order was entered into the medical record of an older adult patient, who is receiving intravenous fluids to treat dehydration resulting from gastroenteritis. "Intravenous fluids at 125 mL/hr for 48 hours." The prescriber is contacted regarding which missing aspect of the order?
A. Rate of infusion
B. Volume to be infused
C. Duration of treatment
D. Type of fluids to be infused

____ 10. Which common IV pump setting prevents patients from tampering with the IV rate setting?
A. STOP
B. OFF switch
C. Delete
D. IV lock

11. A patient is to receive amphotericin B, which has been mixed in a 500-mL bag of IV fluid, over 5 hours. What is the flow rate for this infusion? _____ mL/hr

____ 12. A patient with gastroenteritis and dehydration has the following IV order: "1000 mL to infuse IV over 8 hours." Microdrip tubing is available. What is the nurse's best action?
A. Ask the prescriber to clarify the rate in drops per minute.
B. Administer the IV fluids at 125 drops per minute.
C. Ask the prescriber to clarify the type of fluid to be infused.
D. Administer the IV fluid using a controller device at 125 mL/hour.

Antiinfectives: Antibacterial Drugs

chapter

6

LEARNING ACTIVITIES

Identification: Drug Categories

Identify the drug category described.

1. Kills susceptible bacteria by preventing them from forming strong protective cell walls.

    _____

2. Enters bacterial cells and prevents bacteria reproduction by suppressing the actions of enzymes important in making bacterial DNA.

    _____

3. Interferes with bacterial reproduction by preventing the bacteria from making proteins important to their life cycles and infective processes.

    _____

4. Prevents bacteria from making proteins important to their life cycles and infective processes.

    _____

Matching: Bacterial Infection

Match the terms on the right with the descriptions on the left. (Answers may be used only once.)

____ 5. Ability of bacteria to invade and spread

____ 6. Also known as "blood poisoning"

____ 7. Single-celled organisms that have their own DNA

____ 8. Drug that kills bacteria directly

____ 9. Organism that causes infection when the immune system is suppressed

____ 10. Most common cause of death worldwide

____ 11. Organism that does not cause infection or systemic disease

____ 12. Drug that prevents bacteria from dividing and growing

A. Nonpathogenic
B. Bactericidal
C. Infection
D. Bacteriostatic
E. Bacteria
F. Opportunistic organism
G. Sepsis
H. Virulence

Matching: Cell Wall Synthesis Inhibitors

Match the trade or brand names of the following cell wall synthesis inhibitor drugs with their corresponding generic names. (Answers may be used only once.)

_____ 13. Amoxil

_____ 14. Ancef

_____ 15. Azactam

_____ 16. Bicillin CR

_____ 17. Invanz

_____ 18. Keflex

_____ 19. Merrem

_____ 20. Rocephin

_____ 21. Timentin

_____ 22. Vancocin

A. cephalexin
B. ceftriaxone
C. vancomycin
D. aztreonam
E. ticarcillin/clavulanic acid
F. amoxicillin
G. meropenem
H. penicillin G benzathine
I. ertapenem
J. cefazolin

Matching: Protein Synthesis Inhibitors

Match the protein synthesis inhibitor drugs to their corresponding use, action, side effect, precaution, or adverse effect. (Answers may be used only once.)

_____ 23. A parenteral drug that can seriously reduce hearing

_____ 24. Usually prescribed for infections of the skin and respiratory tract in people who are allergic to penicillins and cephalosporins

_____ 25. Can cause significant joint and muscle pain

_____ 26. Enhances the effect of warfarin and greatly increases the risk for bleeding in patients taking both drugs

_____ 27. Can cause severe respiratory depression in infants and children

_____ 28. Has no effect on bacteria that do not require oxygen for survival or metabolism

_____ 29. An oral drug used to treat MRSA

_____ 30. Can cause a permanent gray-yellow staining to tooth enamel if taken during tooth development

A. tetracycline
B. linezolid
C. dalfopristin
D. azithromycin
E. amikacin
F. clarithromycin
G. streptomycin
H. macrolides

Identification: Sulfonamides/Trimethoprim, Fluoroquinolones

Identify whether the actions, uses, side effects, precautions, and adverse effects listed are associated with sulfonamides/trimethoprim or fluoroquinolones.

_____ 31. Tendon rupture

_____ 32. Used to treat and prevent anthrax

_____ 33. Prevent(s) conversion of substances into folic acid

_____ 34. Bactericidal rather than bacteriostatic

_____ 35. Can form crystals in the kidney

_____ 36. Concentrate in urine, causing irritation of nearby tissues

_____ 37. Should not be given to anyone who has a G6PD deficiency

_____ 38. Avoided in infants because severe jaundice is likely to result

_____ 39. Avoided in infants and children because of potential damage to muscle and bone

_____ 40. Used to treat pneumocystis pneumonia

_____ 41. Can be used to treat nonbacterial Infections, such as shigellosis

_____ 42. Works by inhibiting the DNA synthesis of bacteria

Identification: Bacteria

Identify the type of bacteria described.

43. Bacteria that cause infection. _____

44. Nonpathogenic bacteria always present on skin and mucous membranes and in the GI tract.

_____

45. Bacteria that cause disease only in someone whose immune system is not working well.

_____

MEDICATION SAFETY PRACTICE

1. A child weighing 22 pounds is prescribed amoxicillin/clavulanic acid (Augmentin) for otitis media. What is the correct dosage to administer every 8 hours? _____

2. A patient who is allergic to penicillin may also be allergic to _____.

3. A 7-year-old child with a urinary tract infection is prescribed oral trimethoprim/sulfamethoxazole (Bactrim) to take orally. The child weighs 44 pounds. The recommended children's dose based on trimethoprim content is 3-6 mg/kg orally every 12 hours. What is the correct dose for this patient?

_____

4. A patient is taking a sulfonamide drug and has been advised to increase oral fluids. What is the reason these instructions are given?

_____

_____

NEXT-GENERATION NCLEX® EXAMINATION-STYLE CASE STUDY

Scenario: The nurse is administering a patient an intravenous infusion of vancomycin. During the infusion, the patient verbalizes "not feeling right" and demonstrates hoarseness, audible wheezing, and hives around the IV site.

Which intervention(s) should the nurse perform immediately? **Select all that apply.**

_____ A.   Stop the infusion.

_____ B.   Discontinue the IV.

_____ C.   Slow the rate of the infusion.

_____ D.   Ask the patient if they are having difficulty breathing.

_____ E.   Call the Rapid Response Team.

_____ F.   Document the situation.

_____ G.   Reassure the family that the situation is common and not harmful.

_____ H.   Monitor the patient every 15 minutes.

_____ I.   Prepare to give epinephrine and diphenhydramine.

_____ J.   Prepare to give acetaminophen.

PRACTICE QUIZ

_____ 1.   A patient has been prescribed imipenem/cilastatin (Primaxin). For which potential adverse effect of this drug would the nurse monitor?
   A.   Unplanned pregnancy
   B.   Interaction with asthma medication
   C.   Seizures
   D.   "Red man" syndrome

_____ 2.   Which serious adverse effect could occur with vancomycin (Vancocin)?
   A.   Reduced kidney function
   B.   Impaired liver function
   C.   Decreased white blood cell production
   D.   Impaired clotting ability

_____ 3.   A patient is receiving an IV piggyback containing ticarcillin/clavulanic acid (Timentin) and develops difficulty breathing and swelling of the mouth and throat. Which first action would the nurse take?
   A.   Remove the IV access device.
   B.   Notify the prescriber.
   C.   Determine the patient's allergies.
   D.   Stop the infusion of the drug.

_____ 4.   An older adult is prescribed gentamicin. Which nursing assessment is most appropriate to make? *(Select all that apply.)*
   _____ A.   Intake and output
   _____ B.   Appetite
   _____ C.   Bowel elimination
   _____ D.   Hearing ability
   _____ E.   Joint pain

_____ 5.   A patient is taking the oral antibiotic cefdinir (Omnicef) to treat a skin wound infection. Which information is crucial for the nurse to include in patient teaching?
   A.   "This medication may also help your sore throat."
   B.   "If bloody stools develop, contact your prescriber."
   C.   "After your skin infection clears, stop taking the medication."
   D.   "If a vaginal yeast infection occurs, discontinue using this medication."

_____ 6. Ciprofloxacin (Cipro) has been prescribed for a patient who is also taking an antacid. How should the nurse administer these medications?
   A. Omit the prescribed antacid until the ciprofloxacin is no longer necessary.
   B. Administer ciprofloxacin 2 hours before giving the antacid.
   C. Administer ciprofloxacin 2 hours after giving the antacid.
   D. Omit the ciprofloxacin until antacids are no longer necessary.

_____ 7. A patient is taking both a macrolide antibacterial drug and warfarin (Coumadin). The patient should be instructed to observe closely for increased likelihood of which condition?
   A. Coronary thrombosis
   B. Cardiac dysrhythmias
   C. Excessive bleeding
   D. Antibiotic resistance

_____ 8. An older adult is taking levofloxacin (Levaquin) to treat a urinary tract infection. What is the best nursing intervention if this patient develops new onset of pain and inflammation of the Achilles tendon of the heel?
   A. Administer prescribed PRN pain medication.
   B. Assist the patient in learning crutch walking.
   C. Ask the prescriber for a physical therapy consult.
   D. Notify the prescriber of an adverse effect.

_____ 9. Which objective data would the nurse gather that most closely indicates a serious adverse effect of trimethoprim/sulfamethoxazole (Bactrim)?
   A. Increased sun sensitivity
   B. Polycythemia
   C. Skin peeling, sloughing, and blisters
   D. Appearance of thrush in the mouth

_____ 10. A woman who is pregnant asks the nurse midwife to prescribe tetracycline to treat facial acne. She asks why this medication cannot be used during pregnancy. Which is the best response?
   A. Tetracycline can cause a permanent discoloration of the teeth and thin tooth enamel.
   B. Tetracycline can cause damage to the tendons of the developing fetus during pregnancy.
   C. Tetracycline during pregnancy can be associated with allergic responses later in life.
   D. Tetracycline can be resumed once the baby is born, and the mother is breastfeeding.

Antiinfectives: Antiviral Drugs

LEARNING ACTIVITIES

Identification

In the following list of drugs, indicate which might be included in an antiretroviral ART regimen (A), and which would not (NonA).

_____ 1. abacavir (Ziagen)

_____ 2. acyclovir (Zovirax)

_____ 3. amantadine (Symmetrel)

_____ 4. didanosine (ddI, Videx)

_____ 5. zidovudine (Retrovir)

_____ 6. valacyclovir (Valtrex)

_____ 7. oseltamivir (Tamiflu)

_____ 8. emtricitabine (Emtriva)

_____ 9. zanamivir (Relenza)

Matching: Terminology Review

Match the correct definition on the right with its term on the left. (Answers may be used only once.)

_____ 10. Teratogen

_____ 11. Retrovirus

_____ 12. Virulence

_____ 13. Virustatic

_____ 14. Viral load

_____ 15. Common virus

_____ 16. HIV

_____ 17. Opportunistic infection

A. Overgrowth of normally present organisms
B. Number of viral particles in a blood sample
C. Virus that can use either DNA or RNA as its genetic material
D. Organism that causes AIDS
E. An agent that can cause birth defects
F. Measure of how well an organism can invade and grow
G. A virus that uses RNA as its genetic material
H. Drug action that prevents viral growth and reproduction

Matching: Antiviral Drugs

Match each antiviral drug to its corresponding use, action, side effect, precaution, or adverse effect. (Answers may be used only once.)

_____ 18. Highly teratogenic

_____ 19. Administered by oral inhalation only

_____ 20. Dilute parenteral form only with sterile water for injection

_____ 21. Oral suspension requires specific preparation immediately before administration

_____ 22. Has fewer central nervous system side effects than amantadine

_____ 23. Is converted to acyclovir at the cellular level

_____ 24. Can be confused with Zyvox

_____ 25. Can be confused with Valcyte

A. Oseltamivir
B. Relenza
C. Virazole
D. Amantadine
E. Zovirax
F. Rimantadine
G. Valacyclovir
H. Valtrex

Matching: Antiretroviral Drugs

Match each antiretroviral drug or category to its corresponding use, action, side effect, precaution, or adverse effect. (Answers may be used only once.)

_____ 26. Prevents cellular infection by blocking the CCR5 receptor on CD4+ cells

_____ 27. Increase the risk for lactic acidosis in pregnant women

_____ 28. Can be confused with Viracept

_____ 29. Must be given with ritonavir to achieve a high enough blood level to be effective

_____ 30. Is most likely to cause hypersensitivity reactions within the first 4 weeks of therapy

_____ 31. Can only be administered by subcutaneous injection

_____ 32. Should not be administered to any person who is allergic to sulfa drugs

_____ 33. Should not be prescribed for pregnant women if the patient's viral load indicates that traditional ART is effective

_____ 34. Generic names of drugs in this class usually have "vir" in the middle of the name

_____ 35. Can be confused with Retrovir

_____ 36. Patients should avoid taking St. John's wort with any drug from this class

_____ 37. Can be confused with lamotrigine

A. Viramune
B. abacavir
C. darunavir
D. ritonavir
E. NNRTIs
F. Prezista
G. NRTIs
H. maraviroc
I. enfuvirtide
J. raltegravir
K. protease inhibitors
L. lamivudine

Labeling

In the figure below, label the five parts of a common virus.

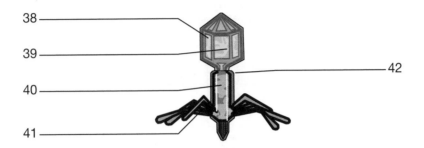

MEDICATION SAFETY PRACTICE

Fill in the blanks with the correct answers.

1. The nurse knows the usual type of tissue through which viruses enter the body is _____ _____.

2. The nurse educates the patient that following a regular schedule is critical in antiviral therapy in order to maintain an adequate _____ _____.

3. Before administering ribavirin (Virazole), the nurse must check the patient's _____ and _____ counts because of the risk for bone marrow suppression.

4. The correct dosage of abacavir (Ziagen) every 12 hours for a child who weighs 44 pounds (20 kg) is _____ mg.

5. Enfuvirtide (Fuzeon) which has not been mixed with water is stored between ____° and ____° F.

6. The nurse monitors for rhabdomyolysis in patients taking raltegravir (Isentress) because the risk is increased when taken with _____-type drugs.

NEXT-GENERATION NCLEX® EXAMINATION-STYLE CASE STUDY

Scenario: A 42-year-old patient is seen in the community clinic for reports of abdominal pain, nausea, and a yellow tinge to the skin. The provider has diagnosed the patient with chronic hepatitis C infection. The provider has prescribed Mavyret (glecaprevir/pibrentasvir), a direct-acting antiviral drug.

For each of the statements made by the patient, specify whether the statement indicates a <u>CORRECT UN-DERSTANDING</u> of the teaching provided, or whether <u>MORE INSTRUCTION IS NEEDED</u> by placing an X in the row next to each statement.

Patient Statement	Correct Understanding	More Instruction Is Needed
"In addition to avoiding alcohol during this treatment phase, I will do my liver a favor and quit drinking altogether."		
"I will avoid sexual intercourse until 1 month after this therapy is completed."		
"If I forget a dose on one day, I will take two doses the next day."		
"When my therapy is completed, I will be immune to being infected with this virus again."		
"If I take this drug at night, I should be sure my stomach is empty."		

PRACTICE QUIZ

_____ 1. A child weighing 66 pounds is to receive amantadine (Symmetrel) orally to treat influenza A. Which dose would the nurse administer every 12 hours?
A. 2.5 mg
B. 30 mg
C. 75 mg
D. 100 mg

_____ 2. Before administering the first dose of valacyclovir (Valtrex) to a patient, the nurse reviews the chart and notes that the patient is also taking phenytoin (Dilantin) for a seizure disorder. The nurse notifies the prescriber because of which action of the antiviral drug?
A. Lowering the seizure threshold
B. Increasing the level of the drug in the blood
C. Reducing the effectiveness of anticonvulsant drugs
D. Causing nausea and vomiting

_____ 3. A 70-year-old patient is taking rimantadine (Flumadine) for treatment of influenza. He calls the clinic to report that he has gained 4 pounds over the weekend, and his ankles are swollen. The patient will need further evaluation for what condition?
A. Lymphedema
B. Pneumonia
C. Heart failure
D. Atrial fibrillation

_____ 4. The nurse would not administer ribavirin (Copegus) for a patient with which condition?
A. Influenza
B. Pregnancy
C. Seasonal allergies
D. Open sores

_____ 5. A diabetic patient on antiretroviral drugs has a marked increase in fasting blood glucose. Which prescription does the nurse anticipate from the provider?
A. A decrease in dosage of the antiretroviral drug
B. An increase in dosage of the antidiabetic drug
C. Beginning administration of a different antidiabetic drug
D. A decrease in the patient's carbohydrate intake

_____ 6. To assess for liver function in patients who are receiving antiretroviral drugs, what should the nurse do daily?
A. Monitor the blood urea nitrogen (BUN) level.
B. Check stool color.
C. Assess the sclera of the eyes.
D. Measure intake and output.

_____ 7. Which statement shows a patient's understanding of the administration schedule of antiretroviral drugs?
A. "I take the pills whenever I wake up in the morning."
B. "If I miss a dose, I don't worry about it."
C. "I have a printed schedule and I follow it closely every day."
D. "When I miss a dose, I just double the amount next time."

_____ 8. Which nursing intervention will be most useful for a patient with peripheral neuropathy as a side effect of antiretroviral drugs?
A. Telling the patient to restrict fluid intake
B. Avoiding apples, prunes, and bran cereal
C. Inspecting feet daily
D. Wearing new shoes until broken in

_____ 9. A 1-year-old child has been diagnosed as being HIV-positive and has been prescribed a nonnucleoside analog reverse transcriptase inhibitor (NNRTI) drug. Which education is included in this patient's plan of care?
A. Children should not receive NNRTIs until age 16.
B. Give this medication with an antacid to decrease nausea.
C. Monitor for anemia by assessing for pallor, fatigue, or cyanosis.
D. If depression develops, St. John's wort is frequently prescribed.

_____ 10. A 27-year-old sexually active woman is taking ribavirin (Copegus, Virazole). Which plan for contraception is appropriate for her?
A. Oral contraception
B. Condoms
C. Intrauterine device
D. Any combination of two methods

11. A patient has been prescribed acyclovir (Zovirax) to treat varicella zoster. The nurse would monitor the patient for which common side effects of acyclovir? *(Select all that apply.)*
_____ A. Liver failure
_____ B. Bone marrow suppression
_____ C. Headache
_____ D. Dizziness
_____ E. Nausea

Antiinfectives: Antitubercular and Antifungal Drugs

LEARNING ACTIVITIES

Matching

Match the possible side effect or adverse effect on the right with the drug listed on the left. (Answers may be used only once.)

____ 1. isoniazid (INH)

____ 2. rifampin (Rifadin, Rimactane)

____ 3. pyrazinamide (PZA)

____ 4. ethambutol (EMB, Myambutol)

A. Optic neuritis
B. Peripheral neuropathy
C. Reddish-orange stain to secretions
D. Increased uric acid formation

Fill in the Blank

5. For ringworm of the scalp, children may be prescribed the drug _____.

6. A patient who is taking isoniazid should avoid _____ to prevent hypertension.

7. A patient's skin and urine may be stained _____ when taking rifampin.

8. Which measures may help to avoid a severe sunburn when taking an antituberculin drug?

   _____

9. The risk for liver toxicity when taking first-line anti-TB drugs is higher in _____ populations.

10. A patient taking terbinafine (Lamisil) has a reduced white blood cell count and is at higher risk for _____.

Matching: Antitubercular Drugs

Match the characteristics, side effects, or precautions associated with the specific antituberculosis drugs. (Answers may be used more than once.)

_____ 11. Important for patients to see an ophthalmologist while taking this drug

_____ 12. Can raise blood pressure to dangerously high levels if taken with caffeine

_____ 13. Can cause breast tenderness in males

_____ 14. Teach patients that this drug colors the urine and other secretions a reddish-orange

_____ 15. Reduces the pH of intracellular fluid inside white blood cells that are infected with the TB bacillus

_____ 16. Can cause peripheral neuropathy, especially in patients who are malnourished

_____ 17. Should not be taken by infants and young children even when they have active tuberculosis

_____ 18. Is only bacteriostatic and must be used in combination with other antituberculosis drugs to be effective

_____ 19. Increases muscle aches and pains

_____ 20. Increased sensitivity to sun and ultraviolet light

_____ 21. May cause loss of appetite, difficulty concentrating, and sore throat

_____ 22. Pregnant women need higher doses of B-complex vitamins while taking this drug

A. ethambutol
B. isoniazid
C. pyrazinamide
D. rifampin

Matching: Antifungal Drugs

Match the trade or brand names of these antifungal drugs with their corresponding generic names. (Answers may be used only once.)

_____ 23. Ancobon

_____ 24. Cancidas

_____ 25. Diflucan

_____ 26. Eraxis

_____ 27. Fungizone

_____ 28. Lamisil

_____ 29. Nizoral

_____ 30. Noxafil

_____ 31. VFEND

A. flucytosine
B. voriconazole
C. caspofungin
D. fluconazole
E. terbinafine
F. ketoconazole
G. anidulafungin
H. amphotericin B
I. posaconazole

MEDICATION SAFETY PRACTICE

1. An older adult who is taking an echinocandin is at increased risk for developing deep vein thrombosis. Which interventions can help prevent this? *(Select all that apply.)*
   ____ A. Heparin drip
   ____ B. Venous sequential compression device
   ____ C. Deep tissue massage to legs
   ____ D. Range-of-motion exercises
   ____ E. Ambulation
   ____ F. Ace bandage wraps to legs
   ____ G. Adequate fluid intake

2. Based on a dosage formula of 4 mg/kg, the correct dose of ketoconazole (Nizoral) for a child who weighs 22 pounds is _____ mg.

3. The correct maximum daily dose for pyrazinamide (PZA) is _____ mg.

4. A patient says she stopped taking her medication to treat tuberculosis after a month, because she stopped coughing up blood. The patient should be instructed to continue taking the drug for how long?

   _____

5. A patient who is taking several first-line drugs to treat tuberculosis says he likes to drink several cans of beer after work every night. He is advised to stop drinking to avoid developing which adverse effect?

   _____

NEXT-GENERATION NCLEX® EXAMINATION-STYLE CASE STUDY

Scenario: A hospitalized patient has recovered from active tuberculosis and is being prepared for discharge. The patient will be responsible for taking ethambutol and isoniazid as prescribed.

Which priority information would the nurse include in the discharge education regarding the prescribed antitubercular drugs? **Select all that apply.**

____ A. Drink a full glass of water with these drugs.
____ B. A B-complex vitamin is needed while taking isoniazid.
____ C. Moderate alcohol use is all right when taking these drugs.
____ D. Do not take any other drugs or supplements without first checking with your provider.
____ E. Continue to take the drugs for at least 6 months or longer, as prescribed.

PRACTICE QUIZ

1. High doses of ethambutol (Myambutol) can cause optic neuritis. What visual changes might this include? *(Select all that apply.)*
   ____ A. Double vision
   ____ B. Red-green color blindness
   ____ C. Reduced visual fields
   ____ D. Reduced color vision
   ____ E. Blurred vision
   ____ F. Reduced central vision

____ 2. Before administering rifampin (RIF) you should assess for an allergy to which substance?
   A. Sulfonamides
   B. Aspirin
   C. Sulfites
   D. Penicillin

_____ 3. Which statement demonstrates that a patient understands the precautions necessary when taking rifampin (RIF) while on oral contraceptives?
   A. "As long as I don't miss any doses, I will be protected."
   B. "My partner will use condoms until I have finished with the drug."
   C. "I will take two oral contraceptive pills a day instead of just one."
   D. "I will use a second method until one month after I finish taking the rifampin."

_____ 4. First-line antitubercular drugs are indicated for which patient?
   A. Pregnant female, to prevent TB infection
   B. Older male taking lipid-lowering drug
   C. Pregnant female with active TB
   D. Nursing mother

5. A patient with coccidioidomycosis has the antifungal drug amphotericin B (Fungizone) prescribed. Which are serious adverse effects of this drug? (Select all that apply.)
   _____ A. Reduced kidney function
   _____ B. Hypercalcemia
   _____ C. Bowel obstruction
   _____ D. Widespread skin flushing
   _____ E. Fever and chills

_____ 6. Before administering an azole antifungal agent, what should the nurse plan to do?
   A. Administer the drug with grapefruit juice.
   B. Administer the drug with a histamine blocker.
   C. Give the drug at a different time as a proton pump inhibitor.
   D. Premedicate the patient with acetaminophen or ibuprofen.

_____ 7. Which patient teaching point is important to include for a patient taking ketoconazole (Nizoral)?
   A. Apply suntan lotion before using tanning beds.
   B. Wear protective clothing when in the sun.
   C. Restrict fluids to decrease the likelihood of kidney impairment.
   D. Apply antiembolism stockings to prevent deep vein thrombosis.

_____ 8. A child with tinea capitis has been prescribed terbinafine (Lamisil). The child should have this drug administered in which manner?
   A. To the scalp
   B. To the feet
   C. In the groin area
   D. Orally

_____ 9. Which diet recommendation is most crucial to provide for a patient who is taking isoniazid, to prevent peripheral neuropathy?
   A. Decrease saturated fats and cholesterol.
   B. Increase the intake of B vitamins.
   C. Eat foods that are higher in iron and calcium.
   D. Decrease foods that contain uric acids.

_____ 10. A patient who is receiving amphotericin B is also receiving intravenous corticosteroids to reduce which possible adverse effect?
   A. Skin itching
   B. Fever and chills
   C. Decreased kidney function
   D. Blood vessel dilation

Drugs for Pain Control, Migraines, and Skeletal Muscle Relaxants

chapter
9

LEARNING ACTIVITIES

Crossword Puzzle: Terminology Review

Complete the puzzle by identifying the key terms that are described.

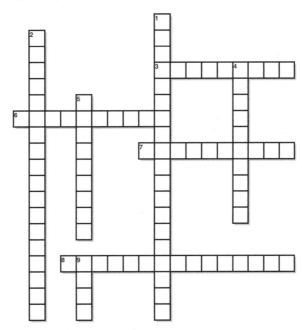

Across
3. The adjustment of the body to long-term opioid use that increases the elimination rate of the drug and reduces the main effects (pain relief) and side effects of the drug
6. Autonomic nervous system symptoms occurring when long-term opioid therapy is stopped suddenly after physical dependence is present
7. Physical changes in autonomic nervous system function that can occur when opioids are used long-term and are not needed for pain control
8. A drug containing any ingredient derived from the poppy plant (or a similar synthetic chemical) that changes a person's perception of pain and has a potential for psychological or physical dependence (two words)

Down
1. A drug containing ingredients known to be addictive that is regulated by the Federal Controlled Substances Act of 1970 (two words)
2. A drug that reduces a person's perception of pain; it is not similar to opium and has little potential for psychological or physical dependence (two words)

4. Drugs of any class that provide pain relief either by changing the perception of pain or by reducing its source
5. The psychologic need or craving for the "high" feeling that results from using opioids when pain is not present
9. An unpleasant sensory and emotional experience associated with acute or potential tissue damage; it is whatever a patient says it is and exists whenever a patient says it does

Matching

Match the statements about types of pain on the left with the terms on the right. (Answers may be used only once, and not all options may be used.)

_____ 1. Physical changes in the autonomic nervous system function that can occur when opioids are used long-term and are not needed for pain control.

_____ 2. The psychological need or craving for the "high" feeling that results from using opioids when pain is not present

_____ 3. The point at which pain is perceived

_____ 4. The adjustment of the body to long-term opioid use that reduces the pain relief of the drug

_____ 5. Autonomic nervous system symptoms occurring when long-term opioid therapy is stopped suddenly after physical dependence is present

A. Tolerance
B. Addiction
C. Dependence
D. Withdrawal
E. Pain threshold
F. Pain tolerance

Identification: Types of Pain

For each pain characteristic listed, label as "A" for acute pain or "C" for chronic pain.

_____ 6. Often has an identifiable cause

_____ 7. Exact cause may or may not be known

_____ 8. Pain may be described as burning, aching, or throbbing

_____ 9. Pain may be described as sharp, stabbing, or pricking

_____ 10. Improves with time

_____ 11. Does not improve with time, and may even worsen

_____ 12. Unlimited duration

_____ 13. Limited duration

_____ 14. Triggers physiologic responses such as increased heart rate and breathing

_____ 15. Physiologic responses go away over time

MEDICATION SAFETY PRACTICE

For each statement below, label the drug as Schedule I, II, III, or IV, and provide one example of a drug in that schedule.

_____ 1. Accepted for medical use in the U.S. and has a low potential for abuse compared to drugs in other schedules.

_____ 2. A high potential for abuse, but is accepted for use as a treatment in the U.S. However, abuse may lead to severe psychological or physical dependence.

_____ 3. Currently accepted for treatment in the U.S., and the potential for abuse is lower than most of the drugs in other schedules. However, abuse may lead to moderate or low physical dependence or high psychological dependence.

_____ 4. The lowest potential for abuse compared to drugs in other schedules, and may be found in cough and antidiarrheal preparations.

_____ 5. Not accepted for medical use in treatment in the U.S. and has a high potential for abuse.

Briefly answer each question after reading the scenario below.

A patient has been prescribed morphine for postoperative pain control. The patient calls the nurse to ask for pain medication, and states that the pain rating is at "8." His last dose of pain medication was 6 hours ago.

6. Before administering the drug, which two physical assessment parameters are most important for the nurse to assess?

7. The patient states, "That pain medicine really knocks me out! But it sure helps with the pain." What information is most important to teach the patient at this time?

8. The medication order reads, "morphine, oral solution (Roxanol), 15 mg every 4 hours, PO, as needed for pain." The medication is available in a unit-dose solution of 10 mg/5 mL. How many mL will the nurse administer for the ordered dose? _____ mL

NEXT-GENERATION NCLEX® EXAMINATION-STYLE CASE STUDY

Scenario: The patient is a 28-year-old woman who has migraine headache pain for an average of 20 days per month. Her only other health problem is asthma for which she uses a prevention inhaler (Advair) twice daily. She tries to swim for an hour three times weekly for exercise. She is now prescribed rimegepant 75 mg orally every other day to prevent or reduce her incidence of migraine headaches. The nurse is developing a teaching plan with take-home instructions/precautions about this drug.

Use an X to indicate which patient statements indicate a <u>CORRECT UNDERSTANDING</u> of therapy with rimegepant and which statements indicate <u>MORE INSTRUCTION NEEDED</u>.

Patient Statements	Correct Understanding	More Instruction Needed
"If I develop a migraine on a day when I have already taken a dose for prevention, I will wait 2 hours to repeat the dose."		
"If I lose more than 2 lb in a week, I will notify my prescriber."		
"Even though I love grapefruit juice, I will not drink it on the days I take the drug."		
"If I have nausea and am unable to keep an oral dose of the drug down, I will go to the prescriber to get an injection of the drug."		
"I will test my facial muscles daily, especially around my eyes, to make sure they are not weaker or won't work."		
"I will drink plenty of water and take a stool softener daily to prevent constipation."		

PRACTICE QUIZ

1. Which factors may reduce a patient's pain tolerance? *(Select all that apply.)*
   ____ A. Fear
   ____ B. Distraction
   ____ C. Lack of sleep
   ____ D. Relaxation
   ____ E. Anxiety

____ 2. A patient who is experiencing chronic pain would likely experience which symptoms?
   A. Burning, aching, or throbbing pain
   B. Pain felt superficially on the body
   C. Increased heart rate and blood pressure
   D. Sweating and increased respiratory rate

3. A patient will be receiving extra-strength acetaminophen (Tylenol) for pain following hernia surgery. Which conditions would the nurse be concerned about?? *(Select all that apply.)*
   ____ A. Liver disease
   ____ B. History of alcoholism
   ____ C. Arthritis
   ____ D. Hypothyroidism
   ____ E. Kidney disease

_____ 4. A patient states, "I've had this pain for almost a year and my doctor told me I need to take an antidepressant. What's that for? I'm not depressed!" Which response by the nurse is most appropriate?
A. "Maybe you really are depressed and just not aware of it."
B. "Your doctor is concerned you might be addicted to pain medication."
C. "Antidepressants help increase the amount of endorphins in the brain."
D. "You have likely developed a tolerance to effects of pain medications."

_____ 5. A patient is receiving an opioid drug through patient-controlled analgesia. Which patient assessment, is of most concern?
A. A sleeping patient who wakes up when called by name
B. Reports of nausea
C. Respiratory rate of 8 breaths per minute
D. Oxygenation saturation of 96% on room air

_____ 6. A patient reports feeling nauseated after taking an oral opioid for pain. Which nursing action is most appropriate?
A. Instruct the patient to take the medication with food.
B. Tell the patient that the nausea will pass after a few doses.
C. Ask the prescriber to order the opioid in an intravenous form.
D. Provide the patient with a low-fiber diet.

_____ 7. A 5-year-old child reports pain after a tonsillectomy, saying "My throat really hurts." The child is to receive opioids. When medicating this patient, which nursing intervention is most appropriate?
A. Use the FLACC scale to determine the child's relative pain intensity.
B. Recognize that many surgical procedures are not as painful for children as for adults.
C. Observe for the common side effect of diarrhea, and administer antidiarrheals as needed.
D. Use an apnea monitor, pulse oximetry, and frequent assessments after medicating the child.

_____ 8. A patient has ingested a large amount of acetaminophen. Which medication will the nurse administer to prevent liver damage?
A. Acetylcysteine
B. Naloxone
C. Naltrexone
D. Hydromorphone

_____ 9. A patient has received a parenteral dose of hydromorphone. Thirty minutes later, the patient's respiratory rate is 8 breaths per minute, and the patient is extremely drowsy. Which nursing action would the nurse perform first?
A. Assess the patient's blood pressure.
B. Gently shake the patient's arm.
C. Squeeze the patient's trapezius muscle.
D. Apply firm pressure to the nail bed.

_____ 10. A patient is taking an extended-release (ER) dose of hydrocodone to treat cancer pain. The patient is advised to change positions slowly to avoid which common side effect?
A. Drug tolerance
B. Respiratory depression
C. Hallucinations
D. Orthostatic hypotension

_____ 11. A patient with chronic pain has difficulty swallowing tablets and capsules and would also like to avoid injections for as long as possible. Which drug is available as a lollipop?
A. Oxycodone
B. Tramadol
C. Fentanyl
D. Meperidine

12. Which nursing interventions are appropriate to take after administering an opioid drug to a patient who has sustained a fractured humerus? *(Select all that apply.)*
    ____ A. If the patient's respiratory rate is 14/min, awaken the patient by calling his or her name.
    ____ B. Warn the patient that pupil dilation is common while taking this category of drugs.
    ____ C. Have naloxone (Narcan) available in the emergency cart in the event a reversal is needed.
    ____ D. Remind the patient to call for help before getting out of bed to ambulate.
    ____ E. Place side rails up and the call light within easy reach of the patient.

____ 13. Which drug is most likely prescribed to treat a patient's pain and burning from diabetic neuropathy?
    A. Acetaminophen (Tylenol)
    B. Pregabalin (Lyrica)
    C. Ibuprofen (Motrin, Advil)
    D. Oxycodone (Percodan)

____ 14. These medications are in the narcotics storage unit. Which one has the highest potential for abuse?
    A. Fentanyl
    B. Tylenol No. 4
    C. Tramadol (Ultram)
    D. Cough syrup with codeine

General Antiinflammatory Drugs

LEARNING ACTIVITIES

Identification: Infection or Inflammation?

For the following, place an X in the appropriate column (Infection or Inflammation) that matches the characteristics of each description.

		Infection	Inflammation
1.	Normal reaction of the body to injury or invasion		
2.	Invasion of the body by microorganisms		
3.	Allergic reactions (hay fever, asthma)		
4.	Nonspecific (same tissue response for any location or cause)		
5.	Manifests with sprained joints and blisters		
6.	Greater risk occurs when a person takes systemic corticosteroids		

Multiple Response

7. Which are common side effects or adverse effects of corticosteroids? *(Select all that apply.)*
   ____ A. Sodium and fluid loss
   ____ B. Hypertension
   ____ C. Excessive sleeping
   ____ D. Nervousness
   ____ E. Weight loss
   ____ F. Moon face
   ____ G. Buffalo hump
   ____ H. Fragile skin
   ____ I. Excessive muscle strength
   ____ J. Thickened scalp hair

8. Which are signs and symptoms of acute adrenal insufficiency? *(Select all that apply.)*
   ____ A. Confusion
   ____ B. Muscle weakness
   ____ C. Rapid irregular pulse
   ____ D. Nausea and vomiting
   ____ E. Salt craving
   ____ F. Weight loss

Matching: Drug Types

Match each term with its corresponding definition. (Answers may be used only once; not all options may be used.)

____ 9.   Antihistamines

____ 10. Antiinflammatory drugs

____ 11. Corticosteroids

____ 12. Disease-modifying antirheumatic drugs
          (DMARDs)

____ 13. Nonsteroidal antiinflammatory drugs
          (NSAIDs)

A. Prevent or limit inflammation by slowing or
    stopping inflammatory mediator production
B. A chemical that binds to receptor sites and
    causes inflammatory responses
C. Prevent or limit the tissue and blood vessel
    responses to injury or invasion by slowing
    the production of one or more inflammatory
    mediators
D. Reduces the progression and tissue destruc-
    tion of the inflammatory disease process by
    inhibiting tumor necrosis factor
E. Prevents inflammatory mediator histamine
    from binding to its receptor site
F. Drugs that prevent or limit inflammatory
    responses to injury or invasion

Matching: Inflammatory Response

Match the characteristics associated with stages I, II, or III of the inflammatory response. (Answers may be used more than once.)

____ 14. Lasts until healing is complete.

____ 15. Mediators are released that make blood vessels dilate and be-
          come leaky.

____ 16. Characterized by redness, swelling, and pain.

____ 17. Begins at the initial injury but may not be evident until the exu-
          date stage is over.

____ 18. Characterized by increased secretions.

____ 19. May be accompanied by a low-grade fever.

____ 20. Known as the stage of tissue repair.

____ 21. Many new cells come to the area and release more mediators.

____ 22. Known as the exudate stage.

____ 23. Begins within minutes after the injury or invasion and lasts for
          hours.

____ 24. Cells are stimulated to divide and form scar tissue.

____ 25. Known as the vascular stage.

A. Stage I
B. Stage II
C. Stage III

Matching: Nonsteroidal Antiinflammatory Drugs

Match the trade or brand names of the following NSAIDs with their corresponding generic names. (Answers may be used only once.)

_____ 26. Ibuprofen

_____ 27. Naproxen

_____ 28. Celecoxib

_____ 29. Oxaprozin

_____ 30. Aspirin

_____ 31. Piroxicam

_____ 32. Indomethacin

_____ 33. Nabumetone

_____ 34. Meloxicam

_____ 35. Diclofenac

A. Indocin
B. Motrin
C. Ecotrin
D. Celebrex
E. Relafen
F. Aleve
G. Daypro
H. Feldene
I. Cambia
J. Mobic

Fill in the Blank

36. During stage _____ of the inflammatory response, the nurse would expect to see large numbers of white blood cells in the patient's complete blood count.

37. Exudate (tissue drainage) is also commonly referred to as _____

38. Patients may lose function when damaged tissues are replaced with _____ tissue.

39. The nurse would teach the patient who is to receive adalimumab (Humira) how to give an injection by the _____ route

40. A patient with severe _____ _____ should not receive DMARDs.

MEDICATION SAFETY PRACTICE

1. All of the NSAIDs except aspirin can reduce blood flow to which organ? _____

2. Which NSAID is recommended for children? _____

3. Compared to the recommended adult dose of cetirizine (Zyrtec), the common dose for children is _____.

4. A child weighing 35 pounds has an IM injection of methylprednisolone (Solu-Medrol) 30 mg prescribed. Does this fall within the recommended range? Why or why not?

5. A patient is to receive prednisone 10 mg PO at 8 AM. The medication tray is supplied with prednisolone 20-mg scored tablets. What action would the nurse take?

6. Several patients will be receiving an initial injection of a DMARD in the clinic today. What safety precautions should be in place? What is a common problem with the site of injection of a DMARD?

NEXT-GENERATION NCLEX® EXAMINATION-STYLE CASE STUDY

Scenario: The nurse is preparing to administer an antihistamine via the intravenous (IV) route to an older adult patient who experienced urticaria and dyspnea due to an allergic reaction. The nurse notes the patient has a history of asthma but is not on maintenance therapy. Recent vital sign measurements are: T 98.2° F; P 65; R 12; and BP 124/76.

Highlight or underline the elements in the paragraph above that the nurse would consider before giving the IV antihistamine to the patient.

PRACTICE QUIZ

____ 1. A community health educator is discussing aspirin use. Which instruction is most appropriate regarding aspirin use in children?
   A. It is frequently used to prevent febrile seizures in children with influenza.
   B. It is contraindicated in children due to the risk of developing Reye's syndrome.
   C. It is recommended to treat fever and discomfort caused by chickenpox.
   D. It is associated with Reye's syndrome, a form of renal failure.

2. Which are common assessment findings for a patient who has used corticosteroids for several months? *(Select all that apply.)*
   ____ A. Decreased facial hair
   ____ B. Decreased waist circumference
   ____ C. Increased fat distribution between shoulders
   ____ D. Muscle wasting
   ____ E. Abdominal striae

____ 3. A patient taking corticosteroids should have which instruction included in patient teaching to avoid stomach ulcers?
   A. Take the medication just before bedtime.
   B. Take the medication by injection.
   C. Take the medication on an empty stomach.
   D. Take the medication with food.

____ 4. The nurse would instruct male patients to use antihistamines with caution due to the risk of which side effect?
   A. Confusion
   B. Hypertension
   C. Urinary retention
   D. Nausea

____ 5. A patient who is taking an antihistamine that causes drowsiness must be taught that additional drowsiness may result if the medication is combined with which element?
   A. Carbohydrate-rich meal
   B. Green leafy vegetables
   C. Alcoholic beverages
   D. Grapefruit juice

____ 6. An older adult patient who is taking corticosteroids for severe arthritis is looking forward to a visit from her preschool-aged grandchildren. The nurse would teach the patient about the patient's higher risk of which condition while taking corticosteroids?
   A. Infection
   B. Muscle atrophy
   C. Weight changes
   D. Nausea and vomiting

____ 7. A patient with diabetes is prescribed corticosteroids for asthma. The patient will require additional monitoring for which condition?
   A. Abdominal striae
   B. Weight loss
   C. Increased blood glucose
   D. Fluid retention

____ 8. A patient with a sprained ankle asks why the ankle is swollen. What would be the nurse's best response?
   A. "Infection is occurring in the injured area."
   B. "Your blood vessels are constricting which causes the swelling."
   C. "The capillaries leak fluid into the tissues when there is an injury."
   D. "Your body is not making enough white blood cells."

____ 9. A patient taking 50 mg of celecoxib (Celebrex) for arthritis pain should be instructed to immediately report which occurrence to the prescriber?
   A. Bruising
   B. Gum bleeding
   C. Anorexia
   D. Chest pain

____ 10. A patient who is taking a COX-1 NSAID is scheduled for surgery in a week. What is the patient at increased risk for?
   A. Bleeding
   B. Infection
   C. Nausea
   D. Deep vein thrombosis

____ 11. The nurse will be administering a daily NSAID to a patient. When is the best time to administer this medication?
   A. Between meals
   B. Anytime
   C. With meals or milk
   D. At bedtime

____ 12. The nurse would monitor a patient taking a leukotriene inhibitor for which common side effect?
   A. Headache
   B. Hives
   C. Liver impairment
   D. Anaphylaxis

Immunizations and Immunosuppressant Drugs

chapter
11

LEARNING ACTIVITIES

Matching: Terminology Review

Match each definition with the corresponding term. (Answers may be used only once; not all options may be used.)

_____ 1. Type of antibody-mediated immunity a person has if antibodies made by another person against an antigen are injected into the body

_____ 2. Vaccine composed of science-made substances that are very similar to the parts of a virus or bacterium that causes disease

_____ 3. A vaccine composed of organisms that could cause diseases but have been killed or inactivated by heat, radiation, or chemicals

_____ 4. Vaccine that contains live organisms that have been modified so they are no longer capable of causing disease

_____ 5. The type of antibody-mediated immunity that is started when a person is invaded by a foreign organism without assistance, and B cells learn to make antibodies against the invaders

_____ 6. Type of antibody-mediated immunity started when an antigen is deliberately placed into the body to force B cells to make a specific antibody against it

_____ 7. A vaccine that contains either a modified toxin that an organism produces or an actual part of the organism

_____ 8. Type of antibody-mediated immunity acquired as a result of antibodies transferred to a fetus or infant from the mother through the placenta and through breast milk

_____ 9. A type of biologic drug composed of antibodies targeted against specific proteins that cause tissue damage

_____ 10. Laboratory-generated pieces of genetic material that code for making a specific part of an organism

A. Artificially acquired active immunity
B. Monoclonal antibodies
C. Toxoid
D. mRNA vaccines
E. Artificially acquired passive immunity
F. Naturally acquired passive immunity
G. True immunity
H. Inactivated vaccine
I. Attenuated vaccine
J. Biosynthetic vaccine
K. Naturally acquired active immunity

Fill in the Blank

11. A human will not develop distemper because of _____ immunity.

12. Any cell, product, or protein with a code different than your own that enters your body and is recognized by the immune system as foreign is a(n) _____ to you.

13. _____ and _____ are examples of attenuated vaccines.

14. The nurse should teach a person who travels to an area of the world where contagious diseases are more common to receive specific vaccinations against _____, _____, _____, and _____.

15. A patient believes she has been exposed to chickenpox but does not remember if she had the disease as a child. The patient can have a(n) _____ _____ blood level drawn to determine if she is protected against the disease.

16. Disease-modifying antirheumatic drugs (DMARDs) reduce disease progression and tissue destruction by inhibiting _____ _____ _____.

17. _____ _____ act by purposely destroying cells.

18. Mycophenolate reversibly inhibits a(n) _____ needed for lymphocyte reproduction and prevents T-cells already present from being active.

19. Polyclonal antibodies are produced by other animals, such as _____ and _____.

20. All selective immunosuppressants can cause the patient to be at an increased risk for _____.

21. The pharmacy employee who is mixing antiproliferative drugs is using personal protective equipment because the drug can be absorbed through _____ and _____ _____.

MEDICATION SAFETY PRACTICE

1. Which vaccines would a pregnant woman *not* receive?

2. A child who has undergone a kidney transplant is to receive azathioprine (Imuran) 2 mg/kg orally every day. The child weighs 78 pounds. How much of the drug should the nurse administer per dose?

3. Which organ system may fail due an antiproliferative drug?

4. Which equipment should be nearby when monoclonal or polyclonal antibodies are being administered? Why?

5. A patient has undergone a liver transplant. Which four areas of instruction should the nurse provide to maintain the effectiveness of the immunosuppressant drugs?

6. Which instructions are most crucial to provide for a patient taking sirolimus or cyclosporine?

NEXT-GENERATION NCLEX® EXAMINATION-STYLE CASE STUDY

Scenario: An 82-year-old patient with a history of rheumatoid arthritis presents to the emergency department with swollen joints, T 101.8° F, and severe abdominal pain. The patient stated that she is taking Xeljanz 11 mg twice daily for her rheumatoid arthritis. She also states she has a rash on her back and is very nauseated. Her husband asks if his wife can have her breakfast tray which includes toast, milk, grapefruit juice, bacon, and fruit cup.

Highlight or underline the findings in the paragraph above that are related to major complications of JAK inhibitors and are of immediate concern to the nurse.

PRACTICE QUIZ

____ 1. A patient taking oral sirolimus has been provided instructions on how to take the medication. Which patient statement indicates the need for further instruction?
   A. "I can disguise the flavor of this medication by mixing it with grapefruit juice."
   B. "I can take this medication with a meal if needed to prevent stomach upset."
   C. "If I take this medication at 8 AM, I can take the cyclosporine at 1 PM."
   D. "I should follow the mixing instructions on the label provided by the pharmacist."

____ 2. A woman who had an organ transplant is taking an antiproliferative agent, and is now considering having a child. Which patient instruction is most important for the nurse to provide?
   A. "You are not as likely to reject the new organ while you are pregnant."
   B. "You should use two reliable methods of contraception while on this drug."
   C. "If you do get pregnant, consider breastfeeding to provide immunity to the baby."
   D. "If you stop taking the medications, you may begin your pregnancy right away."

____ 3. Which diseases are most likely to be treated with DMARDs? *(Select all that apply.)*
   ____ A. Crohn's disease
   ____ B. Peptic ulcers
   ____ C. Pseudomembranous colitis
   ____ D. Psoriatic arthritis
   ____ E. Ankylosing spondylitis

____ 4. Which immunizations would an older adult receive? *(Select all that apply.)*
   ____ A. Measles
   ____ B. Pneumonia
   ____ C. Shingles
   ____ D. Seasonal influenza
   ____ E. Polio

____ 5. A parent brings a 2-week-old infant to the pediatrician and says, "I've been worried about the pertussis outbreak. When is the earliest my baby should get the pertussis vaccine?" Which would be the nurse's answer?
   A. "It can be given today."
   B. "When the baby is 1 year old."
   C. "When the baby is 6 months old."
   D. "When the baby is 2 months old."

____ 6. Which is an example of a toxoid vaccine?
   A. Rubella
   B. Measles
   C. Tetanus
   D. Chickenpox

_____ 7. Which type of immunity does breastfeed-
ing provide to an infant?
   A. Naturally acquired active immunity
   B. Naturally acquired passive immunity
   C. Artificially acquired active immunity
   D. Artificially acquired passive
       immunity

_____ 8. At age 11, a patient contracted measles
when his brothers and sisters also had
the disease. Which type of immunity
provides this patient with long-lasting
immunity?
   A. Naturally acquired active immunity
   B. Naturally acquired passive immunity
   C. Artificially acquired active immunity
   D. Artificially acquired passive
       immunity

_____ 9. In a clinic that provides immunizations,
the nurse finds a vial of last year's flu
vaccine that is not expired. Why wouldn't
the nurse administer it to a patient in the
current year?
   A. The expiration dating system is
       not accurate and is not likely to be
       reliable.
   B. A new vaccine is developed annually
       for viruses predicted to be prevalent
       this year.
   C. Last year's vaccine would likely
       cause a very severe drug allergy or
       anaphylaxis.
   D. Third-party insurers will not cover
       vaccines that should have been given
       last year.

_____ 10. A patient is taking a calcineurin inhibitor
drug. The nurse will monitor the patient
for liver toxicity by assessing which sign?
   A. Redness of the conjunctival sac
   B. Cloudiness over the pupils of the eye
   C. Yellowing of the sclera of the eye
   D. Purulent drainage mixed with tears

_____ 11. A patient taking polyclonal antibod-
ies should be questioned about aller-
gies to which animal prior to taking the
medication?
   A. Birds
   B. Cats
   C. Horses
   D. Dogs

Drugs That Affect Urine Output

chapter **12**

LEARNING ACTIVITIES

Matching

Match the correct category of drug on the right with the name of the drug on the left. (Answers may be used more than once.)

_____ 1. oxybutynin (Detrol)

_____ 2. solifenacin (Vesicare)

_____ 3. hydrochlorothiazide (Microzide)

_____ 4. torsemide (Demadex)

_____ 5. metolazone (Zaroxolyn)

_____ 6. spironolactone (Aldactone)

_____ 7. furosemide (Lasix)

_____ 8. trospium chloride (Sanctura XR)

_____ 9. darifenacin (Enablex)

_____ 10. bumetanide (Bumex)

_____ 11. ethacrynic acid (Edecrin)

A. Diuretic
B. Urinary antispasmodic

Fill in the Blank

Fill in the blanks for each question with the correct answers.

12. A natriuretic diuretic is one that causes excretion of _____ and _____ in the urine.

13. The part of the kidney where filtration takes place is the _____.

14. The detrusor muscle squeezes urine from the _____ into the _____.

15. Diuretics should be taken in the morning to decrease the incidence of _____.

16. The patient taking potassium-sparing diuretics should be aware of these signs of an increased potassium level: _____, _____, _____, and _____.

MEDICATION SAFETY PRACTICE

_____ 1. How long will the nurse take to administer furosemide IV 40 mg?
   A. 2 minutes
   B. 4 minutes
   C. 20 minutes
   D. 40 minutes

_____ 2. Which beverage should a patient taking bumetanide (Bumex) avoid?
   A. Grapefruit juice
   B. Milk
   C. Wine
   D. Green tea

_____ 3. A patient taking a loop diuretic should report which symptom as an early indication of ototoxicity?
   A. Decreased urine output
   B. "Ringing" in the ears
   C. "Popping" sounds in the ears
   D. Hearing voices no one else can hear

_____ 4. Which fall prevention intervention would the nurse include in the plan of care for a patient taking a potassium-sparing diuretic?
   A. Assist the patient to move slowly from a sitting to a standing position.
   B. Leave oranges, bananas, and grapefruit close within the patient's reach.
   C. Discuss the possibility of vest restraint devices with the health care provider.
   D. Suggest the patient remain in bed while taking this medication.

_____ 5. A patient is taking oxybutynin gel packets to treat overactive bladder. The nurse would advise her to avoid which activity?
   A. Walking too far away from a bathroom
   B. Taking the medication at night
   C. Exercising in hot, humid weather
   D. Using the topical gel on the upper arms

NEXT-GENERATION NCLEX® EXAMINATION-STYLE CASE STUDY

Scenario: A 74-year-old patient was admitted to the hospital for possible heart failure. The patient is reporting shortness of breath and swelling of the lower legs. The nurse assesses that the patient has diffuse crackles in the lower lung fields on auscultation and 3+ pitting edema of the lower extremities. O_2 sat is 86% on room air. The provider has prescribed furosemide 40 mg IV now, then furosemide 20 mg po daily.

Which instructions are important for the nurse to provide to this patient about taking furosemide? **Select all that apply.**

_____ A. "I will monitor your blood pressure regularly while you are taking this medication."
_____ B. "The provider has ordered that you can get up as needed, so you don't need to call for assistance before getting out of bed."
_____ C. "You will need to weigh weekly while on this medication."
_____ D. "If you notice any changes in your hearing, be sure to report it."
_____ E. "You may have to lower the volume on your television while on this medication."
_____ F. "Be sure to report any new-onset muscle weakness."
_____ G. "Take your dose late in the evening so your sleep will not be affected."
_____ H. "It is important for us to monitor your potassium and sodium levels daily."

PRACTICE QUIZ

____ 1. A patient taking a potassium-sparing diuretic should be monitored for which side effect?
   A. Gynecomastia
   B. Alopecia
   C. Hypertension
   D. Hyperglycemia

____ 2. A patient is being evaluated for treatment with hydrochlorothiazide (Microzide). For which laboratory value would the nurse notify the prescriber?
   A. Urine specific gravity of less than 1.0028
   B. Serum white blood cell (WBC) count greater than 4000/mm^3
   C. Potassium below 3 mEq/L
   D. Serum creatinine of 1 mg/dL

____ 3. Which question would the nurse ask when assessing a patient who is taking bumetanide (Bumex) in combination with gentamicin (Garamycin)?
   A. "What is the date today?"
   B. "How many fingers do you see?"
   C. "Can you hear this whisper?"
   D. "Can you touch your index finger to your nose?"

____ 4. Which statements best demonstrate a patient's understanding of treatment with tolterodine (Detrol)? *(Select all that apply.)*
   ____ A. "I need to decrease my fluid intake while I am on this medication."
   ____ B. "My husband is going to drive until I see how this drug will affect me."
   ____ C. "I will change the patch every day."
   ____ D. "I will call the doctor if I get a rash where the patch has been."
   ____ E. "This drug will help stop the sudden need to go that I've been having."

____ 5. A patient is taking 20 mg of metolazone (Zaroxolyn) by mouth daily to reduce edema. The nurse will provide which patient education? *(Select all that apply.)*
   ____ A. Slowly change positions from lying to sitting and sitting to standing.
   ____ B. Limit fluid intake to 1 liter per day.
   ____ C. Increased saliva production can be managed by reducing water intake.
   ____ D. Wear sunscreen and appropriate clothing to avoid sunburn.
   ____ E. Use caution in tasks that require mental activity and muscle strength.

____ 6. What instruction should be given to a patient who is taking hydrochlorothiazide (Microzide) and potassium when nausea develops?
   A. "Hold the potassium until the nausea is over."
   B. "Take the medication with food to avoid nausea."
   C. "Decrease the amount of potassium to every other day until you feel better."
   D. "Decrease the amount of diuretic and the amount of potassium by one-half for one day."

____ 7. An older adult is taking furosemide (Lasix). Which special precautions are necessary for this patient? *(Select all that apply.)*
   ____ A. Report new onset of muscle weakness to the prescriber.
   ____ B. Elevated potassium levels may result from this medication.
   ____ C. Instruct the patient to sit on the side of the bed before standing up.
   ____ D. Hearing loss and tinnitus can be associated with the use of furosemide.
   ____ E. Older adults are less sensitive to the effects of furosemide.

_____ 8. Which advice would the nurse give to a pregnant woman regarding thiazide diuretics?
   A. The medication can cause increased fetal potassium levels.
   B. The medication can be taken to lower blood pressure during pregnancy.
   C. It is best to wait until breastfeeding to resume taking this medication.
   D. This medication is associated with jaundice in the newborn.

_____ 9. Which instruction would the nurse provide to a patient who has diabetes while taking furosemide (Lasix)?
   A. Eat an additional 300-500 calories a day to avoid blood sugar decreases.
   B. Monitor your blood sugar more closely for an increase.
   C. You may be more sensitive to rapid drops in your blood sugar level.
   D. Your health care provider will likely suggest a decrease in your insulin dose.

_____ 10. Which instruction is important for the nurse to include in patient teaching for an older adult who is taking a loop diuretic?
   A. Avoid fruits such as bananas, oranges, and grapefruit in your diet.
   B. Increase the amount of foods containing fiber to avoid constipation.
   C. You may be at higher risk of falling while taking this medication.
   D. Hearing loss is a common occurrence during aging and is not concerning.

_____ 11. The nurse would advise a female patient who is taking spironolactone (Aldactone) about which common side effect?
   A. Development of hirsutism
   B. Shrinkage of breast tissue
   C. Premenstrual syndrome
   D. Decreased voice loudness

Drug Therapy for Hypertension

chapter
13

LEARNING ACTIVITIES

Matching

Match the correct mechanism of action on the right with its drug classification on the left. (Answers may be used only once.)

_____ 1. Diuretic

_____ 2. Beta blocker

_____ 3. ACE inhibitor

_____ 4. Angiotensin II receptor agonist

_____ 5. Calcium channel blocker

_____ 6. Alpha blocker

_____ 7. Alpha-beta blocker

_____ 8. Central-acting adrenergic agent

_____ 9. Direct vasodilator

A. Combine alpha/beta blocker effects
B. Slow movement of calcium into cells
C. Oppose excitatory effects of norepinephrine at alpha receptors
D. Limit epinephrine activity
E. Stimulate brain alpha receptors
F. Eliminate salt and water from body
G. Cause arterial dilation
H. Block vasoconstrictors
I. Change action of renin-angiotensin-aldosterone system

Fill in the Blank

Fill in the blanks for each question with the correct answers.

10. Diffuse swelling of the face including the eyes, lips, and tongue is a characteristic of
_____.

11. Beta blockers and alpha blockers affect the _____ receptors.

12. Hardening of the arterial walls is characteristic of _____.

13. Orthostatic hypotension manifests within 3 minutes of when a patient
_____.

14. Secondary hypertension is related to specific _____ and
_____.

MEDICATION SAFETY PRACTICE

_____ 1. A patient has forgotten to take a dose of prescribed medication for hypertension. Which would the nurse advise the patient to do?
A. Take double the amount when it is time for the next dose.
B. If the next dose is in less than 4 hours, just skip the dose that was missed.
C. Since the next dose is due in 2 hours, take the missed dose right away.
D. Take the missed dose immediately, and then skip the next scheduled dose.

_____ 2. As a result of reduced fluid volume and relaxation of arteries, most patients taking diuretics are at risk for which side effect?
A. Dehydration
B. Dizziness
C. Dementia
D. Demineralization

_____ 3. Which schedule would be initiated when stopping therapy with beta blockers?
A. Daily
B. Weekly
C. Gradually
D. Immediately

_____ 4. Captopril (Capoten) 25 mg PO is prescribed. The pharmacy sends scored tablets of 12.5 mg. How many tablets should be administered?
A. ½
B. 2
C. 2½
D. 4

_____ 5. Which is the nurse's priority action for a patient who develops angioedema while taking angiotensin-converting enzyme (ACE) inhibitors?
A. Hold the next dose of medication to see if the condition improves.
B. Discontinue the medication and call the prescriber.
C. Administer the medication slowly and observe the patient's reaction.
D. Decrease the dose by one-half to see if the condition improves.

NEXT-GENERATION NCLEX® EXAMINATION-STYLE CASE STUDY

Scenario: An older adult patient is being seen in the family practice clinic for follow-up of primary hypertension and reports a headache. The provider had previously prescribed lisinopril 40 mg and hydrochlorothiazide 25 mg daily. The patient was asked to keep a blood pressure diary and bring that to the clinic. The nurse notes that the patient's average daily blood pressure is 108/64 mm Hg. Vital signs today are BP 150/90 mm Hg, P 110, R 20, T 98.6° F, and O_2 sat of 98%. The patient reports a persistent dry cough that is worse at night and 2+ edema to both lower extremities.

Highlight or underline the data in the scenario above which is relevant for the nurse to notice for a patient taking lisinopril and hydrochlorothiazide for primary hypertension.

PRACTICE QUIZ

____ 1. A patient is taking a calcium channel blocker. Which best describes how this medication lowers blood pressure?
   A. It increases the movement of calcium into the cells of the heart and blood vessels.
   B. It relaxes the body's blood vessels.
   C. It decreases the supply of oxygen-rich blood to the heart.
   D. It limits the activity of epinephrine on the heart and blood vessels.

____ 2. A patient has been taking captopril (Capoten) for several weeks when severe swelling of the lips and difficulty breathing develop. The nurse recognizes this as which adverse effect?
   A. Neutropenia
   B. Photosensitivity
   C. Reactive airway disease
   D. Angioedema

____ 3. After administering losartan (Cozaar), for which condition does the nurse monitor the patient?
   A. Potassium level higher than 5.5 mEq/L
   B. Sodium level of 140 mEq/L
   C. Decreased bowel sounds and constipation
   D. Weight loss and increased urine output

____ 4. Which statement by a patient best indicates a correct understanding of instructions about taking angiotensin-converting enzyme (ACE) inhibitors?
   A. "I'll use a salt substitute to flavor my food."
   B. "After several months I won't need to worry about facial swelling."
   C. "I'll need to use sunscreen and protective clothing for my trip to the beach."
   D. "If I drink alcohol, my blood pressure would likely increase."

____ 5. Which statement made by a pregnant woman taking angiotensin-converting enzyme (ACE) inhibitors is true?
   A. "After delivery, I can use ACE inhibitors and breastfeed."
   B. "ACE inhibitors can cause liver disorders in my baby."
   C. "ACE inhibitors can cause birth defects."
   D. "ACE inhibitors can cause my baby to develop low potassium."

6. A patient who is taking atenolol (Tenormin), a beta blocker, would be monitored for which side effects? *(Select all that apply.)*
   ____ A. Tachycardia
   ____ B. Difficulty breathing
   ____ C. Fever or sore throat
   ____ D. Dizziness when standing up
   ____ E. Hyperkalemia

____ 7. A patient who has been taking a calcium channel blocker would be monitored for which symptom of Stevens-Johnson syndrome?
   A. Hypothermia
   B. Gingival hyperplasia
   C. Gynecomastia
   D. Skin lesions

8. Which medications would the nurse instruct a male patient not to take with drugs for erectile dysfunction? *(Select all that apply.)*
   ____ A. Beta blockers
   ____ B. Alpha-beta blockers
   ____ C. Alpha blockers
   ____ D. Calcium channel blockers
   ____ E. DHT blockers

____ 9. Which drug has been safely used to treat pregnancy-induced hypertension?
   A. Valsartan (Diovan)
   B. Captopril (Capoten)
   C. Methyldopa (Aldomet)
   D. Atenolol (Tenormin)

10. A patient who is taking losartan (Cozaar) is going on a 2-week cruise to the Bahamas during the summer. The nurse would advise the patient to avoid which activities while on the cruise? (*Select all that apply.*)
    ____ A. Sitting for long periods of time
    ____ B. Consuming alcoholic beverages
    ____ C. Exercising on the boat deck
    ____ D. Eating fried or unusually spicy foods
    ____ E. Taking a drug to treat erectile dysfunction

____ 11. A patient who has been taking metoprolol (Lopressor) for several months states, "I've got nothing to live for anymore. I'd be better off if I just died. I'm just depressed all the time." Which would be the nurse's next action?
    A. Discuss the possibility of a dose increase with the prescriber.
    B. Remind the patient of the importance of taking this medication.
    C. Tell the patient to stop taking the medication immediately.
    D. Inform the prescriber of the patient's possible depression symptoms.

____ 12. A patient contacts the clinic at 4 PM on a Friday, saying she has just run out of the prescription for atenolol (Tenormin) which she takes for hypertension. The prescriber has left for the weekend, and the pharmacist will not refill the prescription without a refill authorization for the medication. Which would be the nurse's best action?
    A. Contact the on-call prescriber for a refill authorization.
    B. Report the pharmacist to the state board of pharmacy.
    C. Ask the patient to call the office back first thing Monday.
    D. Ask the patient to remain calm.

Drug Therapy for Heart Failure

chapter

14

LEARNING ACTIVITIES

Fill in the Blank

Fill in the blanks with the correct answers.

1. For a headache related to initial treatment with nitroglycerin, the patient should take _____.

2. Left heart failure is characterized by a dilated or overstretched _____ _____.

3. Decreased renal blood flow related to heart failure is compensated by activation of the _____ _____ _____.

4. Most heart failure begins in the _____ _____.

5. Digoxin increases the force of _____ _____.

Matching: Vasodilators

Match the vasodilator on the left with the correct intended response on the right. (Answers may be used more than once for each vasodilator, and not all options may be used.)

_____ 6. hydralazine (Apresoline)

_____ 7. nitroglycerin

_____ 8. isosorbide (Isordil)

    A. Decreased heart workload
    B. Increased blood pressure
    C. Increased blood flow to coronary arteries
    D. Vasoconstriction of arteries
    E. Increased venous vasodilation
    F. Decreased blood pressure
    G. Increased arterial vasodilation
    H. Decreased blood flow to coronary arteries

Matching: Heart Failure

Match the symptom of heart failure with the appropriate cause. (Answers may be used more than once.)

_____ 9. Shortness of breath

_____ 10. Oliguria during the day

_____ 11. Distended abdomen

_____ 12. Frothy, pink-tinged sputum

_____ 13. Crackles and wheezes

_____ 14. Enlarged liver

A. Right-sided heart failure
B. Left-sided heart failure

MEDICATION SAFETY PRACTICE

Determine whether each statement is True or False. If the statement is False, correct it to make it True.

_____ 1. Previous doses of nitroglycerin ointment should be vigorously rubbed off before administering a new dose.

_____ 2. Nitroglycerin ointment should be kept on the patient's skin around the clock in order to maintain a therapeutic blood level.

_____ 3. Digoxin (Lanoxin) toxicity may be characterized by bradycardia, loss of appetite, and yellow halos appearing around objects.

_____ 4. The trade name for the drug dopamine is Dobutamine.

Solve this problem:

5. Digoxin (Lanoxin) 0.25 mg PO is prescribed. The medication is available in scored tablets of 0.125 mg each. How many pills would the nurse administer? _____

NEXT-GENERATION NCLEX® EXAMINATION-STYLE CASE STUDY

Scenario: The nurse is caring for a patient who has a history of heart failure and hypertension. The patient has recently been prescribed digoxin 5 mcg/kg orally daily.

For each assessment finding below, indicate whether the finding is <u>EXPECTED</u> or <u>REQUIRES FOLLOW-UP</u> by the nurse by placing an X in the appropriate column.

Assessment Finding	Expected	Requires Follow-Up
Dizziness upon standing		
Heart rate of 50		
Blurred vision		
Nausea and vomiting		
Fatigue		
Palpitations		
Digoxin level 1.2 ng/mL		

PRACTICE QUIZ

_____ 1. A patient taking hydralazine (Apresoline) for heart failure has a temperature of 104° F. His white blood cell (WBC) count has dropped from 8000/mm³ to 4000/mm³. What is the patient at risk for experiencing?
A. Bleeding
B. Seizure
C. Infection
D. Falling

_____ 2. A patient on digoxin (Lanoxin) reports feeling tired and nauseated. What is the priority nursing assessment to make?
A. Temperature
B. Urine output
C. Apical pulse
D. Mental status

_____ 3. Before administering nitroglycerin ointment to a patient, what precaution would the nurse take?
A. Putting on a facemask
B. Handwashing with bactericidal solution
C. Putting on a gown
D. Putting on gloves

_____ 4. Which instruction would the nurse give to the patient regarding oral nitroglycerin?
A. "Keep it in the refrigerator."
B. "Store the amber bottle in a dark place."
C. "Keep a drink of water close by so you can swallow the pills quickly in an emergency."
D. "If you do not feel a tingling sensation, the drug is no longer potent."

_____ 5. The nurse is educating a female patient of childbearing age about taking digoxin. Which statement made by the nurse is appropriate?
A. "Drink plenty of water before breastfeeding."
B. "Digoxin passes from the mother to the fetus."
C. "This drug is perfectly safe for your baby."
D. "Try to exercise regularly to reduce the drug's effect on the fetus."

_____ 6. Hydralazine (Apresoline) dosage in children is based on which measurement?
A. Height
B. Age
C. Heart rate
D. Weight

_____ 7. What would be the correct initial dose of nesiritide (Natrecor) for an adult patient with heart failure who weighs 68 kg?
A. 10 mcg
B. 130 mcg
C. 136 mcg
D. 100 mcg

_____ 8. After beginning therapy with IV potassium for heart failure, a patient's cardiac monitor shows an irregular heart rate of 60 beats per minute. The patient reports feeling weak and confused. Which serum potassium range would result from IV potassium therapy (expressed in mmol/L)?
A. 3.5-5.0
B. 1.5-3.0
C. 0.5-1.5
D. 5.2-6.8

_____ 9. Which instruction would the nurse include when teaching a patient about the use of digoxin (Lanoxin)?
A. "If this medication causes an upset stomach, take it with an antacid."
B. "Take your pulse monthly and notify your prescriber if your pulse is less than 60."
C. "Digoxin toxicity is less likely to occur if you are also taking diuretics."
D. "Keep all laboratory appointments for drug level testing."

_____ 10. A patient is undergoing treatment for heart failure with dopamine. The nurse would recognize which condition as a possible side effect of this treatment?
A. The cardiac output is increased.
B. The heart rate lowers 20 beats per minute.
C. The white blood cell count is lowered.
D. Tissue damage occurs if there is infiltration.

11. A patient has received instructions on increasing potassium intake in the diet from the nurse. The patient demonstrates understanding of the instructions by selecting which menu items? _(Select all that apply.)_
_____ A. Tuna sandwich
_____ B. Baked potato
_____ C. Brazil nuts
_____ D. Winter squash
_____ E. Black beans

Drug Therapy for Dysrhythmias

chapter

15

LEARNING ACTIVITIES

Matching

Match the drug on the left with its correct drug category on the right. (Answers may be used more than once.)

_____ 1. lidocaine (Xylocaine)

_____ 2. esmolol (Brevibloc)

_____ 3. tocainide (Tonocard)

_____ 4. propranolol (Inderal)

_____ 5. amiodarone (Cordarone)

_____ 6. diltiazem (Cardizem)

_____ 7. verapamil (Calan)

A. Beta blocker
B. Potassium channel blocker
C. Calcium channel blocker
D. Class 1b sodium channel blocker

Fill in the Blank

Fill in the blanks with the correct answers.

8. The ability of the cardiac muscle cells to fire on their own is known as _____.

9. Before administering atropine (Atropine Sulfate), the nurse must assess for a history of
    _____.

10. To treat digoxin toxicity, a drug is given to bind with the medication and prevent its action. The generic
    and trade names of this drug are _____ and _____.

List the medications that may be given through the endotracheal tube during a cardiac/respiratory emergency when an intravenous line has not been established.

11. _____

12. _____

13. _____

14. _____

15. _____

MEDICATION SAFETY PRACTICE

1. Some of the life-threatening effects of procainamide are _____, _____, _____, and _____.

2. Some serious adverse effects of dofetilide (Tikosyn) are _____ and _____.

3. In addition to signs of thyroid problems, for which effects would a patient taking amiodarone (Cordarone) be monitored?

_____

_____

4. The nurse is administering adenosine (Adenocard). What special injection technique would the nurse use?

_____

5. The nurse instructs a patient who is taking amiodarone (Cordarone) to have eye examinations every 6 to 12 months to assess for _____ _____.

NEXT-GENERATION NCLEX® EXAMINATION-STYLE CASE STUDY

Scenario: Joan Stevens is a 32-year-old woman with a history of atrial fibrillation and premature ventricular contractions (PVCs) who was admitted to the cardiac medical/surgical unit. The provider has prescribed amiodarone 200 mg orally daily. On assessment, the nurse notes that the patient has an irregular apical pulse and edema of the lower extremities. Current lab values are decreased serum T_4, increased liver enzymes, decreased serum potassium, and decreased WBC count. Lung sounds exhibit crackles in both lower lung bases. Today's weight shows an 8-lb increase since admission 2 days ago.

Highlight or underline the information in the scenario above that the nurse should follow up for this patient taking amiodarone.

PRACTICE QUIZ

____ 1. Before beginning treatment with atropine (Atropine Sulfate) for bradycardia, the nurse would assess for a history of which disorder in the patient?
A. Multiple sclerosis
B. Muscular dystrophy
C. Glaucoma
D. Diabetes

____ 2. A patient has been recently prescribed quinidine (Quinaglute). Which statement made by the patient indicates further teaching is required?
A. "I should report any weight gain to my provider."
B. "I will take my medication at the same time every day."
C. "I will avoid drinking milk."
D. "I should take my medication with a citrus fruit like orange."

_____ 3. A patient taking digoxin (Lanoxin) reports a weight gain of 7 pounds in the last week. The nurse would assess the patient for which condition?
A. Pregnancy
B. Clinical depression
C. Bowel obstruction
D. Heart failure

_____ 4. In an emergency, lidocaine (Xylocaine) may be given intravenously or by airway inhalation. Why are these routes of administration used?
A. They avoid interaction with other drugs.
B. They reduce the risk of adverse effects.
C. When given orally, the liver renders the drug ineffective.
D. They are closer to the tissue where drug action is needed most.

_____ 5. Patients who are taking tocainide (Tonocard) may have increased risk of infection because of which adverse effect?
A. Pneumonitis
B. Confusion
C. Neutropenia
D. Hypotension

6. Which drugs are used to treat ventricular dysrhythmias? (Select all that apply.)
_____ A. atropine (Atropine Sulfate)
_____ B. lidocaine (Xylocaine)
_____ C. digoxin (Lanoxin)
_____ D. flecainide (Tambocor)
_____ E. digoxin immune fab (DigiFab)
_____ F. propranolol (Inderal)
_____ G. esmolol (Brevibloc)

_____ 7. A patient is experiencing bradycardia accompanied by symptoms of dizziness. Which medication would be prescribed for this patient?
A. Adenosine
B. Atropine
C. Amiodarone
D. Atenolol

8. What is the correct dose in milligrams of ibutilide (Corvert) for an adult patient who weighs 140 pounds? (The recommended adult dose for a patient weighing less than 60 kg is 0.01 mg/kg over 1 minute; 1 mg for a patient over 60 kg.)
_____ mg

9. An older adult has been given a dose of lidocaine (Xylocaine). Which nursing interventions are important for the nurse to include? (Select all that apply.)
_____ A. Instruct the patient to change positions slowly.
_____ B. Advise the patient to use handrails to reduce the risk for falls.
_____ C. Advise the patient to report episodes of diarrhea.
_____ D. Monitor laboratory results for increased white blood cells.
_____ E. Observe the patient for episodes of confusion.

_____ 10. A patient who has been taking amiodarone (Cordarone) reports difficulty breathing and a cough, which has been present for several weeks. Which nursing action is most appropriate?
A. Report the patient's symptoms to the health care provider.
B. Suggest screening for the possibility of tuberculosis infection.
C. Advise the patient these are common and expected side effects.
D. Teach the patient these side effects usually resolve with time.

_____ 11. A patient who has been taking amiodarone (Cordarone) for several months is discussing a trip to the American southwest during May and June. Which recommendation is most important for the nurse to make?
A. Restrict liquid intake and minimize exposure to heat.
B. It would be better if you stayed at home instead of vacationing.
C. Wear dark sunglasses and protective clothing when outdoors.
D. Ask your provider to temporarily stop the amiodarone while on the trip.

Drug Therapy for High Blood Lipids

LEARNING ACTIVITIES

Crossword Puzzle: Lipid-Lowering Drugs

Complete the puzzle by identifying the correct terms that are described.

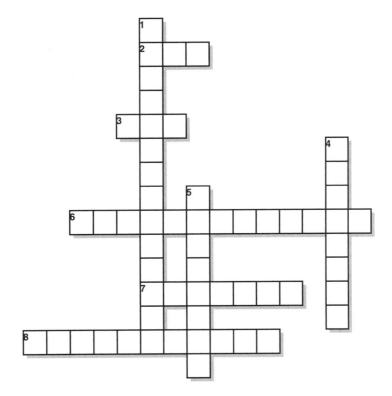

Across
2. "Good" cholesterol in the body (abbreviation)
3. "Bad" cholesterol in the body (abbreviation)
6. Vitamin B that helps decrease cholesterol levels (two words)
7. Drugs that inhibit production of cholesterol
8. Waxy, fatty material in cell walls

Down
1. Muscle cell breakdown
4. Genetic hyperlipidemia
5. Drugs that lower triglycerides

Matching

Match the drug with its appropriate drug category. (Answers may be used more than once.)

_____ 1.   atorvastatin (Lipitor)

_____ 2.   ezetimibe (Zetia)

_____ 3.   niacin extended release (Niaspan)

_____ 4.   pravastatin (Pravachol)

_____ 5.   cholestyramine (Questran)

_____ 6.   gemfibrozil (Lopid)

_____ 7.   fenofibrate (Tricor)

_____ 8.   colestipol (Colestid)

_____ 9.   simvastatin (Zocor)

A.   Bile acid sequestrant
B.   Cholesterol absorption inhibitor
C.   Fibrate
D.   Nicotinic acid
E.   Statin

Fill in the Blank

10. The nurse would teach a patient that the side effect of flushing or hot flashes when taking nicotinic acid (Niacor) can be reduced by taking the drug with _____ or with _____.

11. The nurse teaches a patient with diabetes that nicotinic acid (Niacor) can have the effect of _____ blood glucose levels.

12. Bile acid sequestrant drugs bind cholesterol-containing bile in the _____ and remove them via _____ _____.

13. Cholesterol absorption inhibitors prevent the uptake of cholesterol from the _____ _____ into the _____ _____.

14. _____ primarily lower triglycerides.

15. Statin drugs lower LDL cholesterol and triglycerides by _____ _____ by the body.

MEDICATION SAFETY PRACTICE

1. Before beginning therapy with lipid-lowering drugs, the patient must have baseline testing done for _____ function.

2. Statins should not be given to patients who drink more than _____ alcoholic beverages a day.

3. Fibrates can increase the effectiveness of warfarin (Coumadin) and cause a prolonged _____ time.

4. Gemfibrozil (Lopid) may interact with statin drugs by interfering with their _____.

5. A patient has been taking rosuvastatin (Crestor) for several months to lower the cholesterol level. Today the patient reports having abdominal pain under the ribs on the right side and having darker urine and lighter gray stools. What is the likely explanation for this?

    _____

    _____

6. In the above situation, what would be the nurse's next action?

    _____

    _____

NEXT-GENERATION NCLEX® EXAMINATION-STYLE CASE STUDY

Scenario: Joseph Page is a 64-year-old male with a prior history of a heart attack. When discharged from the hospital after treatment for the heart attack, the patient was given prescriptions for cholestyramine 10 g orally with meals and warfarin 2.5 mg orally daily. The provider also advised Mr. Page to take 81 mg of aspirin daily. Mr. Page is now visiting his primary care provider for follow-up.

For each lab result below, indicate whether the result is <u>EXPECTED</u> for a patient taking cholestyramine or <u>REQUIRES FOLLOW-UP</u> by the nurse to immediately notify the provider by placing an X in the appropriate column.

Lab Result	Expected	Requires Follow-Up
LDL 48 mg/dL		
WBC 10,700 mm^3		
Creatinine 1.1 mg/dL		
INR 4.5		
Total cholesterol 200 mg/dL		
ALT 110 U/L		
Vit D 9 ng/mL		

PRACTICE QUIZ

1. What lifestyle changes are discussed with a patient who is beginning drug therapy for treatment of hyperlipidemia and hypercholesterolemia? *(Select all that apply.)*
    _____ A. Weight control
    _____ B. Ergonomic workstation
    _____ C. Regular exercise
    _____ D. Driving at night
    _____ E. Low-fat diet
    _____ F. Organic diet

2. Although generally safe for older adults, which condition is a contraindication for medication therapy with statins? *(Select all that apply.)*
    _____ A. Diabetes mellitus
    _____ B. Glaucoma
    _____ C. Liver disease
    _____ D. Hypertension
    _____ E. Myopathy
    _____ F. Alzheimer's disease

_____ 3. The nurse instructs the patient to take the tablet form of bile acid sequestrants with at least how many ounces of water?
A. 2-4
B. 6-9
C. 10-12
D. 12-16

_____ 4. Which beverage interferes with the metabolism of fibrates and makes them less effective?
A. Coffee
B. Milk
C. Grapefruit juice
D. Pomegranate juice

5. A patient has been taking nicotinic acid (Niacor) for several months and is now at a dosage of 1 g twice per day. The medication is available in 500-mg tablets. How many tablets per day will the patient take? _____ tablet(s)

_____ 6. Which intervention can reduce the flushing or hot flashes associated with nicotinic acid?
A. Give the drug with estrogen hormone replacement.
B. Administer the drug with acetaminophen (Tylenol).
C. Give the drug with large amounts of fluid.
D. Give the drug during or after a full meal.

_____ 7. A patient who is taking a statin agent should be monitored for which serious adverse effect?
A. Decreased liver function
B. Decreased platelet counts
C. Increased white blood cell counts
D. Hypotension and tachycardia

_____ 8. A patient asks how statin drugs work in the body. What is the nurse's best response?
A. "They bind with cholesterol in the intestine."
B. "They work by controlling the rate of cholesterol produced by the liver."
C. "They reduce the amount of cholesterol absorbed by the body."
D. "They are a type of vitamin B that increases HDL cholesterol."

_____ 9. An older adult taking a statin agent reports suddenly developing muscle aches and weakness. Which is the most important question for the nurse to ask this patient?
A. "Have you taken any over-the-counter NSAIDs?"
B. "Have you noticed any numbness or tingling sensations in your extremities?"
C. "Have you noticed a brownish color to your urine?"
D. "Have you noticed any facial flushing or 'hot flashes'?"

_____ 10. A patient's medication history is carefully reviewed by members of the health care team. The patient is currently taking warfarin (Coumadin). It is not likely this patient will have a bile acid sequestrant prescribed for which reason?
A. The bile acid sequestrant would intensify the effect of warfarin.
B. The bile acid sequestrant needs to be taken with aspirin.
C. The bile acid sequestrant would cause the warfarin to be ineffective.
D. The bile acid sequestrant would lower the overall platelet count.

_____ 11. The nurse would assess a patient who will be taking gemfibrozil (Lopid) for which adverse effect of the drug?
A. Kidney stones
B. Deep vein thrombosis
C. Increased creatinine levels
D. Constipation

Drugs That Affect Blood Clotting

chapter
17

LEARNING ACTIVITIES

Crossword Puzzle: Terminology Review

Complete the puzzle by identifying the correct terms that are described.

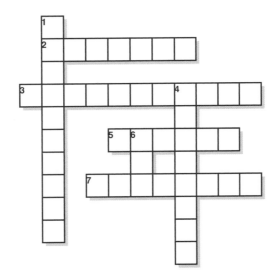

Across
2. Travels through the bloodstream and blocks vessels
3. Process by which blood clots form
5. Protein essence of a blood clot
7. Blood clot in a vessel or the heart

Down
1. Profuse bleeding
4. Converts fibrinogen to fibrin
6. Blood test used to report results of warfarin anticoagulation (abbreviation)

Matching

Match the type of anticoagulant drug on the right with the correct medication names on the left. (Answers may be used more than once.)

_____ 1. darbepoetin alfa (Aranesp)

_____ 2. warfarin (Coumadin)

_____ 3. ticlopidine (Ticlid)

_____ 4. t-PA (Activase)

_____ 5. clopidogrel (Plavix)

_____ 6. tenecteplase (TNKase)

_____ 7. tirofiban (Aggrastat)

_____ 8. reteplase (Retavase)

_____ 9. epoetin alfa (Epogen, Procrit)

_____ 10. eptifibatide (Integrilin)

_____ 11. heparin

_____ 12. oprelvekin (Neumega)

_____ 13. aspirin

_____ 14. enoxaparin (Lovenox)

A. Thrombin inhibitor
B. Clotting factor synthesis inhibitor
C. Antiplatelet
D. Thrombolytic
E. Colony-stimulating factor

Fill in the Blank

15. Clotting factor synthesis inhibitors decrease the production of clotting factors in the _____.

16. _____ drugs break down fibrin in an already-formed clot.

17. Thrombin inhibitors block the action of _____, which converts _____ to _____ to form clots.

18. _____ are drugs that interfere with blood clotting by preventing the activation of platelets.

19. _____ combine with proteins in the plasma to stick together and form a clot.

MEDICATION SAFETY PRACTICE

1. The recommended dose of oprelvekin (Neumega) is 50 mcg/kg once daily. What dose would the nurse give a patient who weighs 154 pounds? _____.

2. Vitamin K is the antidote for _____.

3. Why would the nurse avoid rubbing the injection site after administering subcutaneous heparin?

4. Colony-stimulating factors increase the patient's risk for hypertension, blood clots, strokes, and heart attacks because of increased blood _____ and _____ retention.

5. The nurse carefully reviews the medication history of a patient who takes an anticoagulant drug. Which over-the-counter drugs and herbal supplements would be contraindicated for this patient to take?

6. A patient who is pregnant has a venous thromboembolism. Which medication will most likely be prescribed?

NEXT-GENERATION NCLEX® EXAMINATION-STYLE CASE STUDY

Scenario: A 35-year-old female patient is being seen for a 6-month follow-up at her provider's office after being discharged from the hospital with a diagnosis of deep vein thrombosis. The provider prescribed apixaban (Eliquis) 5 mg orally twice daily. The patient appears short of breath, her face is pale, and she states her arms are itchy. She also states she is having a heavy menstrual period and her gums bled when she brushed her teeth this morning.

Choose the most *likely* options for the information missing from the statement below by selecting from the list of options provided.

The nurse is concerned the patient is having a/an _____1_____ and requires _____2_____.

Options for 1	Options for 2
hemorrhage	epinephrine
heparin-induced thrombocytopenia	vitamin K
anaphylactic reaction	heparin
pulmonary embolism	protamine sulfate

PRACTICE QUIZ

1. Which statement best demonstrates a patient's understanding of how warfarin (Coumadin) works to help after heart valve replacement surgery? *(Select all that apply.)*
   ___ A. "It will thin out my blood so that it won't clot anymore."
   ___ B. "It will make me bruise and bleed more easily, so I must be careful."
   ___ C. "It will dissolve the clots that have formed in my heart."
   ___ D. "New clots will not form as easily in my heart valves."
   ___ E. "Any clots that I still have will not get any bigger."
   ___ F. "I will feel the cold weather more because my blood is thinner now."

___ 2. Which lab tests does the nurse use to determine the effectiveness of heparin administration for a patient who has had a venous thromboembolism (VTE)?
   A. Prothrombin time (PT)
   B. Activated partial prothrombin time (APPT)
   C. Activated partial thromboplastin time (aPTT)
   D. International normalized ratio (INR)

3. A patient who is taking warfarin (Coumadin) therapy is instructed to avoid which foods? *(Select all that apply.)*
   ___ A. Grapefruit
   ___ B. Fava beans
   ___ C. Spinach
   ___ D. Bananas
   ___ E. Kale
   ___ F. Oranges
   ___ G. Broccoli

___ 4. The nurse will administer which medication to a patient on renal dialysis who is anemic?
   A. oprelvekin (Neumega)
   B. alteplase/t-PA (Activase)
   C. clopidogrel (Plavix)
   D. epoetin alfa (Epogen, Procrit)

___ 5. A patient who is taking a clotting factor synthesis inhibitor such as warfarin (Coumadin) would be monitored for which serious adverse effect?
   A. Decreased clotting times
   B. Upset stomach, diarrhea, and fever
   C. Headaches that are severe and will not go away
   D. Increased viscosity of the blood

6. What are important lifespan considerations for an older adult who is taking warfarin (Coumadin)? *(Select all that apply.)*
   ___ A. Aspirin increases the action of warfarin.
   ___ B. Statin drugs decrease the action of warfarin.
   ___ C. Older adults are more likely to develop bruises and bleeding.
   ___ D. Sucralfate (Carafate) increases the effect of warfarin.
   ___ E. Older adults need more frequent monitoring of the international normalized ratio (INR).

___ 7. The nurse would include which important instruction when teaching a patient about colony-stimulating factor therapy?
   A. Tell the patient that weight gain of more than 2 pounds a month should be reported to the prescriber.
   B. Teach the patient how to administer intramuscular injections correctly.
   C. Remind the patient to keep scheduled laboratory appointments for blood tests to monitor therapy.
   D. Instruct the patient to take this medication with adequate amounts of liquid.

___ 8. Several patients are receiving heparin. Which medication would be used as an antidote?
   A. epoetin alfa (Epogen)
   B. enoxaparin (Lovenox)
   C. vitamin K (AquaMEPHYTON)
   D. protamine sulfate

____ 9. Before administering a thrombolytic
drug, the nurse assesses for which abso-
lute contraindication?
A. Chronic peptic ulcer disease
B. Recent spinal or cerebral surgery
C. Blood pressure of 150/92 mm Hg
D. Current use of warfarin (Coumadin)
or aspirin

____ 10. The nurse provides diet instructions to
a patient who will be taking warfarin
(Coumadin) for several weeks. Which
menu selection indicates the need for fur-
ther instruction?
A. Spinach salad with bacon dressing
B. Orange and banana fruit salad
C. Plate of assorted cheeses and grapes
D. Pepperoni pizza and light beer

____ 11. A patient has recently been given an
intravenous injection of heparin. Which
vital sign changes would the nurse report
as signs of a hemorrhage?
A. Increased blood pressure, decreased
pulse
B. Decreased blood pressure, increased
pulse
C. Decreased blood pressure, decreased
pulse
D. Increased blood pressure, increased
pulse

Drug Therapy for Asthma and Other Respiratory Problems

chapter 18

LEARNING ACTIVITIES

Matching: Drug Categories

Match the correct drug category on the right with the correct medication names on the left. (Answers may be used more than once.)

_____ 1. beclomethasone (QVAR)

_____ 2. albuterol (Proventil)

_____ 3. theophylline (Theo-Dur)

_____ 4. triamcinolone (Azmacort)

_____ 5. salmeterol (Serevent)

_____ 6. fluticasone (Flovent)

_____ 7. ipratropium (Atrovent)

_____ 8. budesonide (Pulmicort)

_____ 9. formoterol (Foradil)

_____ 10. omalizumab (Xolair)

_____ 11. tiotropium (Spiriva)

_____ 12. cromolyn

_____ 13. dupilumab (Dupixent)

A. Short-acting beta$_2$ agonist
B. Long-acting beta$_2$ agonist
C. Cholinergic antagonist
D. Methylxanthine
E. Inhaled corticosteroid
F. Mast cell stabilizer
G. Leukotriene inhibitor
H. Biologic

Matching: Terminology Review

Match the term on the right with its correct description on the left. (Answers may be used only once.)

_____ 14.	Air sacs in the lungs where oxygen moves into the blood	A. Lumen
_____ 15.	Airway obstruction disease caused by constriction and inflammation	B. Alveoli
		C. Bronchitis
_____ 16.	A class of complex antiinflammatory drugs derived from living sources	D. Asthma
		E. Mucolytic
_____ 17.	Sound of air moving through narrowed airways	F. Emphysema
_____ 18.	Drug that reduces the thickness of mucus	G. Wheeze
_____ 19.	Open center of a hollow airway	H. Bronchodilator
_____ 20.	Inflammation of the airways	I. Bronchoconstriction
_____ 21.	Disease where the elasticity of alveoli is greatly reduced	J. Biologics
_____ 22.	Tightening of pulmonary smooth muscle, resulting in narrowed airways	
_____ 23.	Drug that relaxes the smooth muscle around airways, causing the center openings to enlarge	

Matching: Pathophysiology of Asthma and COPD

Indicate which characteristics are associated only with asthma, which are associated only with COPD, and which are common to both. (Answers may be used more than once.)

_____ 24.	Involves the airways and the alveoli	A. Asthma
_____ 25.	Causes reduced oxygenation	B. COPD
_____ 26.	Is a reversible condition of airway obstruction	C. Both
_____ 27.	Wheezing	
_____ 28.	Increased size of mucus-producing cells	
_____ 29.	Caused by a combination of bronchitis and emphysema	
_____ 30.	Reduces peak expiratory flow rate (PEFR)	
_____ 31.	No symptoms present between attacks	
_____ 32.	Lumen size is reduced	
_____ 33.	Can be caused by constriction of bronchiolar smooth muscle alone	
_____ 34.	Airway inflammation	
_____ 35.	Loss of elastic tissue in walls of the alveoli	

Fill in the Blank

36. A common method to measure airway function is _____

    _____ _____ _____

    (_____).

37. A patient can use a(n) _____ _____ when about to start an activity that is likely to induce an asthma attack.

38. List four systemic effects of bronchodilators.

39. _____ or _____ _____ can occur if excessive amounts of bronchodilator drugs reach the blood.

40. A child who takes a(n) _____ _____ _____ close to bedtime may have difficulty sleeping.

MEDICATION SAFETY PRACTICE

1. Asthma medication that is used only during an acute episode is known as a(n) _____ drug.

2. A patient just took a short-acting inhaler drug. Which symptoms of an adverse effect would the nurse report immediately to the prescriber?

3. The nurse would ensure that the patient using an oral inhaler knows the proper technique for using it, and for a(n) _____, if one is ordered.

4. If a patient is taking more than one type of inhaled drug, the _____ drug would be given at least 5 minutes before the other drug.

5. A PEFR value that has dropped below 50% indicates what is occurring?

NEXT-GENERATION NCLEX® EXAMINATION-STYLE CASE STUDY

Scenario: Mr. Simmons is seen in Urgent Care for dyspnea related to asthma. Mr. Simmons does not have a primary care provider or take any medications for asthma. On assessment, the nurse notes that his breath sounds are diminished and bronchial wheezing is present. Mr. Simmons' O_2 saturation is 90% via pulse oximetry. The nurse places O_2 at 2 L via nasal cannula per protocol and notifies the provider of Mr. Simmons' status. The provider orders salmeterol nebulizer treatment. After the nebulizer treatment, vital signs are BP 160/100 mm Hg, P 115, R 18, O_2 sat is 96%, and temp is 101.4° F orally.

Indicate which of the patient's symptoms are an <u>INDICATION</u> for, <u>ADVERSE EFFECT</u> of, or <u>UNRELATED</u> to salmeterol by placing an X in the appropriate column for each symptom.

Symptoms	Indication	Adverse Effect	Unrelated
T 101.4° F			
Bronchial wheezing			
O_2 sat 90%			
BP 160/100 mm Hg			
P 115			
R 18			

PRACTICE QUIZ

____ 1. The nurse would assess symptom severity in a patient with asthma or chronic bronchitis by using which method?
   A. FEV_1
   B. PEFR
   C. PEEP
   D. CPAP

____ 2. A patient is taking ipratropium (Atrovent), and reports having difficulty emptying his bladder. Which action would the nurse take?
   A. Report symptoms of kidney disease to the prescriber.
   B. Encourage the patient to drink more fluids.
   C. Ask the prescriber for an order for an indwelling catheter.
   D. Discuss the patient's symptoms with the prescriber.

____ 3. Which important point should be included when teaching patients about the use of long-acting beta$_2$-adrenergic agonists?
   A. "Use this medication whenever you have new symptoms of wheezing."
   B. "Take an extra dose of this medication if your symptoms worsen."
   C. "Take this medication even when symptoms are not present."
   D. "Omit your daily dose of this medication if you are wheezing."

____ 4. A child with asthma is having difficulty using a "rescue" aerosol inhaler effectively. Which alteration in treatment would the nurse discuss with the provider?
   A. Switching the route of administration to oral
   B. Using a nebulized form of the drug with a facemask
   C. Switching to a dry powder inhaler
   D. Changing to a long-acting inhaler

____ 5. What are common side effects associated with inhaled antiinflammatory drugs? *(Select all that apply.)*
   ____ A. Bad taste
   ____ B. Mouth dryness
   ____ C. Seizures
   ____ D. Leukopenia
   ____ E. Oral infection

____ 6. Before administering an inhaled corticosteroid, it is important for the nurse to take which action?
   A. Teach the patient how to use the inhaler or spacer.
   B. Teach the patient to expect nervousness after using.
   C. Prime a new canister of nedocromil (Tilade) once before use.
   D. Administer inhaled corticosteroid agents before bronchodilators.

____ 7. What important instruction would the nurse give to a patient who is taking guaifenesin (Mucinex)?
   A. "This medication is given to treat acetaminophen overdose."
   B. "This medication will thin your mucus and make it easier to cough up."
   C. "This medication can cause an oral infection called *thrush*."
   D. "This medication is used with a nebulizer facemask."

____ 8. A patient has just taken a short-acting inhaler drug to treat asthma symptoms. Which best condition indicates the medication has been effective?
   A. An increase in the respiratory rate
   B. A pulse oximetry value of 85%
   C. An increase of 15% in the peak flow
   D. Wheezing within 2 hours of use

____ 9. A patient has been given instructions on the use of a dry-powder inhaler. Which patient action indicates the need for further instruction?
   A. The patient exhales deeply into the inhaler after the treatment.
   B. The patient stores the device in a dry place, at room temperature.
   C. The patient states she knows not to shake the inhaler prior to use.
   D. The patient removes the inhaler from her mouth as soon as she has inhaled.

____ 10. A patient is using an aerosol inhaler without a spacer. Two puffs are prescribed. How far apart should the puffs be administered?
   A. 10 seconds
   B. 30 seconds
   C. 60 seconds
   D. 120 seconds

____ 11. Which action by the nurse is appropriate during intravenous administration of treprostinil (Remodulin) for a patient with pulmonary hypertension?
   A. Disconnect the intravenous line when assisting the patient to the bathroom.
   B. Utilize strict sterile technique when preparing and administering the drug.
   C. Connect intravenous antibiotic drugs to the same line to prevent needle pain.
   D. Monitor the patient's laboratory tests for signs of deteriorating kidney function.

____ 12. Which is the most important point to include in patient teaching for a female patient with pulmonary hypertension who will have bosentan (Tracleer) prescribed?
   A. "We can electronically transfer this prescription to your retail pharmacist."
   B. "A yellowish tinge to your skin is common while taking this medication."
   C. "If you have any difficulty swallowing the tablet, cut it in half."
   D. "Your pregnancy test must be negative before this drug can be given."

Drug Therapy for Gastrointestinal Problems

LEARNING ACTIVITIES

Matching: Terminology Review

Match the definitions on the right with their correct terms on the left. (Answers may be used only once.)

____ 1. Antiemetic
____ 2. Chemoreceptor
____ 3. Constipation
____ 4. Diarrhea
____ 5. Emesis
____ 6. Mechanoreceptors
____ 7. Nausea
____ 8. Peristalsis
____ 9. Retching
____ 10. Vestibular apparatus
____ 11. Vomiting

A. Frequent watery bowel movements
B. Act or results of vomiting
C. Tension receptors in the bowel that initiate vomiting
D. Forcing stomach contents up through the esophagus and out of the mouth
E. Urge to vomit
F. Labored respiration with the contraction of the abdomen, chest wall, and diaphragm
G. Sensory nerve cells responding to intestinal chemical stimuli and toxins
H. Inner ear structures associated with balance and position sensing
I. Bowel movements that are infrequent and difficult or painful
J. Mass movements in the colon
K. Drugs that prevent or control nausea

Matching: Drugs for Gastrointestinal Problems

Match the drug category on the right with the correct drug names on the left. (Answers may be used more than once.)

____ 12. docusate (Colace)
____ 13. loperamide (Imodium)
____ 14. prochlorperazine (Compazine)
____ 15. bismuth subsalicylate (Pepto-Bismol)
____ 16. meclizine (Dramamine)
____ 17. difenoxin with atropine (Motofen)
____ 18. lactulose (Cephulac)
____ 19. diphenoxylate with atropine (Lomotil)
____ 20. bisacodyl (Dulcolax)
____ 21. calcium polycarbophil (FiberCon)
____ 22. scopolamine (L-hyoscine)
____ 23. granisetron (Kytril)
____ 24. metoclopramide (Reglan)
____ 25. castor oil (Emulsoil)

A. Antidiarrheal drug
B. Antiemetic drug
C. Drug for constipation

Matching: Drugs for Nausea and Vomiting

Match the type of action with the corresponding antiemetic drug. (Answers may be used only once.)

_____ 26. Block dopamine receptors to inhibit one or more vomiting reflex pathways

_____ 27. Inhibit vomiting reflex pathways to stop intestinal cramping and inhibit vestibular input

_____ 28. Block the action of histamine at the H_1 receptor sites, which results in depression of inner ear excitability and reduces vestibular excitability

_____ 29. Bind to and block serotonin receptors in the intestinal tract, which results in blockage of at least two pathways of the vomiting reflex

_____ 30. Directly block dopamine from binding to receptors in the chemotrigger zone and the intestinal tract so that food moves along the intestinal tract more rapidly

A. Dopamine antagonists
B. Antihistamines
C. 5HT3-receptor antagonists
D. Anticholinergics
E. Phenothiazines

Fill in the Blank

31. A(n) _____ drug treats diarrhea by slowing down peristalsis in the gastrointestinal tract.

32. A dopamine antagonist binds to receptors in the _____ _____.

33. A lubricant is a(n) _____ or _____ substance that can help make bowel movements easier.

34. By adding fluid to stool, _____ _____ make bowel movements easier.

35. An antihistamine drug works against nausea/vomiting by blocking the action of histamine at the _____ _____ _____.

36. _____ _____ _____ are drugs that work against nausea and vomiting caused by chemotherapy treatments.

MEDICATION SAFETY PRACTICE

1. A patient is to receive 35 mg of promethazine (Phenergan) IM. The vial that is available contains 50 mg/mL. How many mL of promethazine will the nurse administer to the patient? _____ mL

2. List three causes of constipation.

3. List five symptoms of neuroleptic malignant syndrome.

4. A patient who lives in a hot, humid environment would be advised that taking an antinausea drug such as _____ can cause anticholinergic effects leading to a decrease in sweating, and an increased risk of overheating the body.

5. List three symptoms of Reye's syndrome.

NEXT-GENERATION NCLEX® EXAMINATION-STYLE CASE STUDY

Scenario: Laura Miller is a 45-year-old mother of four who presents to the emergency department with reports of nausea, vomiting, and diarrhea for the past 3 days. The patient also reports feeling very lethargic.

Below is a list of available medications in the patient's chart. **Choose the most *likely* options for the information missing from the table below by selecting from the lists of options provided.**

Medication	Dose, Route, Frequency	Drug Class	Indication
Metoclopramide	10 mg by mouth before meals and at bedtime	3	Gastroesophageal reflux, diabetic gastroparesis
Methylcellulose	1 tbsp in 8 oz of water 2-3 times a day	Bulk forming	4
1	20 g dissolved in 8 oz of liquid daily	Osmotic laxative	Chronic constipation
Difenoxin with atropine	2	Antimotility	Diarrhea

Options for 1	Options for 2	Options for 3	Options for 4
Docusate sodium	25 mg orally PRN every 6 hours	Osmotic laxative	Diarrhea
Promethazine	2 tablets orally, then 1 tablet orally PRN	Stimulant	Constipation
Cyclizine	12.5 to 25 mg orally four times a day	Antiemetic	Bowel motility
Polyethylene glycol	1 mg orally twice daily	Antacid	Nausea

PRACTICE QUIZ

____ 1. Which drug is likely to be most helpful in controlling nausea and vomiting in a patient receiving chemotherapy?
A. Metoclopramide (Reglan)
B. Trimethobenzamide (Tigan)
C. Scopolamine (L-hyoscine)
D. Ondansetron (Zofran)

____ 2. Which drug for the control of nausea and vomiting is contraindicated in a patient who has a history of depression?
A. Promethazine (Phenergan)
B. Prochlorperazine (Compazine)
C. Scopolamine (L-hyoscine)
D. Metoclopramide (Reglan)

____ 3. The nurse would monitor which laboratory result after continued administration of promethazine (Phenergan) or prochlorperazine (Compazine)?
A. Blood urea nitrogen (BUN)
B. Complete blood count (CBC)
C. International normalized ratio (INR)
D. Activated partial thromboplastin time (aPTT)

____ 4. An older adult woman who has problems with constipation wants to know which drug is safe for her to take on a daily or alternate-day schedule. Which drug will most likely be recommended by the health care provider?
A. Polyethylene glycol (MiraLax)
B. Castor oil (Emulsoil)
C. Sodium phosphate (Fleet Enema)
D. Psyllium (Metamucil)

____ 5. A patient with diabetes is advised to take a laxative every other day if no bowel movement occurs. Which laxative is contraindicated for this patient?
A. Bisacodyl (Dulcolax)
B. Lactulose (Cephulac)
C. Polyethylene glycol (MiraLax)
D. Magnesium hydroxide (Milk of Magnesia)

____ 6. The nurse would monitor an older adult who is taking an antiemetic drug for which side effects? *(Select all that apply.)*
____ A. Confusion
____ B. Shuffling gait
____ C. Diarrhea
____ D. Excessive drooling
____ E. Trembling

____ 7. Which statement indicates the patient has understood how to achieve the best response from medications for chemotherapy-induced nausea?
A. "I will take an antiemetic medication 30 minutes before meals."
B. "I will take this medication every night with a small glass of wine."
C. "I will take this medication within 1 hour after chemotherapy begins."
D. "The lip-smacking and tongue movements I am experiencing are expected effects."

____ 8. After administering a medication for diarrhea to a patient, which action is appropriate for the nurse to perform?
A. Instruct the patient to restrict oral fluids.
B. Remind the patient to decrease his or her activity level.
C. Assess the patient for abdominal distention.
D. Assess the patient's fasting blood sugar.

____ 9. A patient who experiences toxic megacolon after taking antimotility drugs would exhibit which signs and symptoms? *(Select all that apply.)*
____ A. Bradycardia
____ B. Fever
____ C. Abdominal pain
____ D. Distended abdomen
____ E. Hypervolemia

_____ 10. A patient is very nauseated immediately after surgery. Which is a dangerous direct complication of this?
    A. Increased risk for aspiration pneumonia
    B. Increased risk for fluid volume overload
    C. Excessive scar tissue from surgical incision
    D. Risk for development of venous thromboembolism

_____ 11. A patient is undergoing chemotherapy and has been experiencing nausea and vomiting with each session. Which instruction given by the nurse is most appropriate to help prevent future nausea events?
    A. "Avoid chemotherapy treatments due to the severity of nausea and vomiting."
    B. "Take the prescribed antiemetic prior to arrival for chemotherapy treatments."
    C. "Let us know once you become nauseated, so we can give you antiemetic medication."
    D. "Nausea and vomiting are seldom associated with chemotherapy treatments."

_____ 12. A patient who frequently experiences motion sickness will be taking meclizine (Antivert) prior to airplane travel. The patient would be instructed about which common side effect of the medication?
    A. Constipation
    B. Involuntary muscle movements
    C. Drowsiness
    D. Abdominal pain

Drug Therapy for Gastric Ulcers, Reflux, and Inflammatory Bowel Disease

chapter

20

LEARNING ACTIVITIES

Matching: Terminology Review

Match each description on the right with its correct term on the left. (Answers may be used only once.)

____ 1.   Antacids
____ 2.   Barrett's esophagus
____ 3.   Dyspepsia
____ 4.   Lower esophageal sphincter (LES)
____ 5.   Esophagogastroduodenoscopy (EGD)
____ 6.   Gastroesophageal reflux disease (GERD)
____ 7.   Gastric ulcer
____ 8.   *Helicobacter pylori*
____ 9.   H$_2$ blocker
____ 10. Peritonitis
____ 11. Regurgitation
____ 12. Immunomodulators

A.   Indigestion
B.   Open sore in the stomach lining
C.   Upper endoscopy exam of the esophagus, stomach, and small intestine
D.   Complication of severe chronic GERD
E.   Esophageal irritation due to stomach acid backing up
F.   Drugs that block the effects of histamine
G.   Backward flow of stomach contents
H.   Inflammation of the abdominal cavity
I.   Bacteria that cause gastric inflammation
J.   Drugs that neutralize stomach acids
K.   Drugs that affect the functioning of the immune system
L.   Muscular ring located where the esophagus joins the stomach

Multiple Choice

____ 13.   What percentage of people in the U.S. are infected with the *Helicobacter pylori* bacteria?
   A.   5-10%
   B.   10-15%
   C.   15-20%
   D.   20-30%

____ 14.   Of the following causes of gastric ulcers, which one is primary?
   A.   Stress
   B.   Diet
   C.   Excess gastric acid
   D.   *H. pylori*

____ 15.   Which weakened sphincter muscle causes GERD?
   A.   Anal
   B.   Upper esophageal
   C.   Pyloric
   D.   Lower esophageal

16. Which dietary factors contribute to reflux? *(Select all that apply.)*
    ____ A. Caffeine
    ____ B. Nicotine
    ____ C. Chewing gum
    ____ D. Chocolate
    ____ E. Black pepper
    ____ F. Alcohol
    ____ G. Red meats
    ____ H. Peppermint
    ____ I. Small meals
    ____ J. Leafy green vegetables
    ____ K. Eggs

Fill in the Blank

17. When _____ _____ exceeds mucus production, the risk for ulcers increases.

18. List four symptoms of a gastric ulcer. _____

    _____

    _____

    _____

19. Usually, the pain of a peptic ulcer is located between the _____ and

    _____.

20. _____ _____ after a meal may prevent irritation of the esophagus associated with GERD.

21. Chronic GERD can lead to serious complications such as _____

    _____ and _____ _____.

Matching: Types of Drugs for PUD and GERD

Match the type of drug used for peptic ulcer disease (PUD) and GERD with its action. (Answers may be used only once.)

____ 22. Decrease the secretion of gastric acid

____ 23. Block the secretion of gastric acid

____ 24. Form a thick coating that covers an ulcer to protect it from further damage

____ 25. Neutralize stomach acid

____ 26. Increase lower esophageal sphincter tone and help empty the stomach

____ 27. Treat *H. pylori* infections

A. Cytoprotective drugs
B. Proton pump inhibitors
C. Histamine H_2 blockers
D. Antibiotics
E. Antacids
F. Promotility drugs

MEDICATION SAFETY PRACTICE

1. Patients taking large doses of antacids containing calcium or aluminum salts over a long period of time are at risk for developing _____.

2. Patients taking Milk of Magnesia for indigestion over a long period of time are likely to develop _____.

3. Antacids such as Alka-Seltzer or Bromo-Seltzer are contraindicated for patients who have _____ _____.

4. Bismuth subsalicylate (Pepto-Bismol) is contraindicated in children because of the risk for developing _____ _____.

5. A patient is to take 15 mL of Maalox at bedtime. What is the household equivalent of this dose? _____

NEXT-GENERATION NCLEX® EXAMINATION-STYLE CASE STUDY

Scenario: Mrs. Stevens was diagnosed with Crohn's disease 2 years ago and has since been taking olsalazine (Dipentum) daily. She is in the clinic today for a routine follow-up and the nurse assesses her health history and lab results.

Which assessment findings by the nurse indicate that the patient is experiencing side effects and/or adverse effects from taking this drug? **Select all that apply.**

_____ A. Increased diarrhea
_____ B. Elevated creatinine level
_____ C. Severe fatigue
_____ D. Rash
_____ E. Migraines
_____ F. Constipation
_____ G. Feeling ill
_____ H. Dizziness
_____ I. Hypoglycemia
_____ J. Muscle pain

PRACTICE QUIZ

1. Which lab tests are monitored for patients who are taking nizatidine (Axid) or cimetidine (Tagamet)? *(Select all that apply.)*
_____ A. Complete blood count
_____ B. Liver function tests
_____ C. Electrolytes
_____ D. Urinalysis
_____ E. Pulmonary function tests

2. A 14-year-old patient who weighs 143 pounds is prescribed clarithromycin (Biaxin) for *H. pylori* infection. The recommended children's dose is 15 mg/kg orally in 2 divided doses. What is the correct dose in milligrams for *each* of the doses given in one day? _____ mg

3. Long-term use of proton pump inhibitors can lead to which conditions? *(Select all that apply.)*
   ____ A. Gastric infections
   ____ B. Bowel obstruction
   ____ C. Drowsiness
   ____ D. Anemia
   ____ E. Halitosis

____ 4. Which statement demonstrates a patient's understanding of therapy with cytoprotective drugs for treatment of GERD?
   A. "I will take this medicine until it relieves my symptoms."
   B. "This drug will be a lifelong treatment for my stomach problems."
   C. "I need to keep my vegetable and fruit intake down while I'm on this medication."
   D. "I must take this drug for as long as my doctor prescribes it."

____ 5. During a follow-up assessment of a patient taking metoclopramide (Reglan) for treatment of GERD, the nurse observes an elevated temperature, respiratory distress, tachycardia, diaphoresis, and urinary incontinence. Which is the priority nursing action for this situation?
   A. Check the patient's medical record for drug allergies.
   B. Notify the prescriber.
   C. Give the antidote for metoclopramide.
   D. Place the patient on a cooling blanket.

____ 6. An older adult has been prescribed cimetidine (Tagamet). Which is a lifespan consideration for this patient?
   A. A black tongue or bowel movement is a common effect of this medication.
   B. Due to decreased calcium absorption, hip fractures are more common.
   C. Older adults are more likely to experience dizziness and confusion.
   D. This patient should be taught how to avoid excessive exposure to the sun.

____ 7. A patient asks how the proton pump inhibitor lansoprazole (Prevacid) will help the symptoms of GERD. Which is the nurse's best response?
   A. "It prevents stimulation of the pumps in your stomach that produce acid."
   B. "It blocks the action of acid-secreting cells in your stomach."
   C. "It neutralizes acids in your stomach to decrease irritation."
   D. "It coats the mucosal lining of your stomach."

____ 8. Which patient statement best indicates a correct understanding of why the antibiotic clarithromycin (Biaxin) has been prescribed along with another medication for ulcers?
   A. "It treats infection with *H. pylori*."
   B. "It is effective against inflammation in the stomach."
   C. "It prevents peritonitis in the event of stomach perforation."
   D. "It treats fever associated with neuroleptic malignant syndrome."

____ 9. A patient has been taking metoclopramide (Reglan) for several months to treat GERD. The nurse notes the patient has uncontrolled jerking–type movements of the mouth and face. She is puckering her lips and has rapid movements of the tongue. These symptoms are consistent with the development of which adverse effect of the medication?
   A. Perforation of a peptic ulcer
   B. Neuroleptic malignant syndrome
   C. Tardive dyskinesia
   D. Parkinson's disease

____ 10. An older adult will be taking metoclopramide (Reglan) to treat symptoms of GERD. Which safety instruction is most crucial for the nurse to provide?
   A. "You must stop driving altogether."
   B. "Never eat spicy or greasy foods again."
   C. "This drug may increase your blood pressure."
   D. "Sit up slowly from a resting position."

____ 11. The nurse is assisting a patient to set up a schedule for taking sucralfate (Carafate) to treat an ulcer. Which is the appropriate schedule for this medication?
A. Every 6 hours around the clock
B. One hour before meals and at bedtime
C. An hour after meals and at bedtime
D. With each meal and then at bedtime

____ 12. A patient is taking bismuth subsalicylate (Pepto-Bismol) to treat an ulcer. The patient reports having constipation, gray-black stools, and a gray-colored tongue. What is the most likely explanation of this?
A. These are common side effects of the medication.
B. These indicate nonhealing of the ulcer.
C. These are symptoms of gastrointestinal bleeding.
D. The patient is exceeding the prescribed dose.

Drug Therapy for Diabetes

LEARNING ACTIVITIES

Crossword Puzzle: Terminology Review

Complete the puzzle by identifying the correct terms described in the clues below.

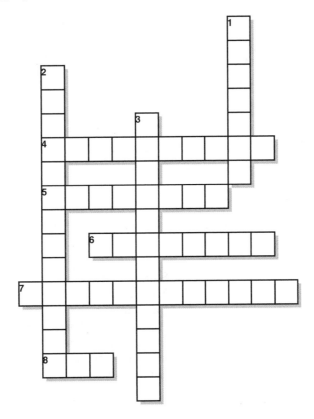

Across
4. Normal range of fasting blood glucose
5. Hormone secreted by pancreas alpha cells
6. Type of diabetes related to reduced insulin effectiveness
7. Excessive byproduct of fat metabolism
8. Body's main chemical energy substance

Down
1. Hormone secreted by pancreas beta cells
2. Higher-than-normal blood glucose level
3. Lower-than-normal blood glucose level

Fill in the Blank

Fill in the blank with the correct term regarding possible complications of poorly controlled diabetes.

1. _____ blood cholesterol levels

2. _____ risk for heart attack

3. _____ wound healing

4. Loss of _____ sensation

5. _____ failure

6. Erectile _____

Fill in the blank with the correct information about the types and durations of insulin.

7. Peak time of insulin aspart (NovoLog) _____

8. Duration of action of regular insulin (Humulin) _____

9. Onset of isophane insulin NPH (Novolin N) _____

10. Duration of action of insulin glargine (Lantus) _____

Matching: Antidiabetic Drugs

Match each type of oral antidiabetic drug on the right with its correct drug name on the left. (Answers may be used more than once.)

_____ 11. pioglitazone (Actos)

_____ 12. glipizide (Glucotrol)

_____ 13. repaglinide (Prandin)

_____ 14. glyburide (DiaBeta, Micronase)

_____ 15. acarbose (Precose)

_____ 16. glimepiride (Amaryl)

_____ 17. nateglinide (Starlix)

_____ 18. glyburide, micronized (Glynase)

_____ 19. metformin (Glucophage)

_____ 20. miglitol (Glyset)

_____ 21. rosiglitazone (Avandia)

_____ 22. exenatide (Byetta)

_____ 23. pramlintide (Symlin)

_____ 24. liraglutide (Victoza)

A. Sulfonylurea
B. Meglitinide
C. Biguanide
D. Alpha-glucosidase inhibitor
E. Thiazolidinedione
F. Incretin mimetic
G. Amylin analogs

Identification: Pathophysiology of Diabetes

Indicate with an X which symptoms, complications, and management strategies are associated with type 1 diabetes, type 2 diabetes, or both type 1 and type 2 diabetes. (Answers will be used more than once.)

Symptom, Complication, and Management Strategy	Type 1 Diabetes	Type 2 Diabetes	Type 1 and Type 2 Diabetes
25. Hyperglycemia is present.			
26. Onset of symptoms is sudden.			
27. Symptoms most commonly begin in adults over age 40.			
28. Always requires insulin for treatment.			
29. The risks for heart disease and kidney disease are increased.			
30. More likely to occur in people who are overweight.			
31. Ketoacidosis is a serious complication.			
32. The most common type of diabetes mellitus.			
33. The patient has an increased risk for infection.			
34. A major symptom before treatment is started is increased thirst.			
35. The patient still makes some of his or her own insulin.			
36. Hypertension is common.			

MEDICATION SAFETY PRACTICE

1. The nurse will instruct a patient to rotate injection sites for insulin to minimize the risk of developing _____ _____.

2. True or False: After inserting the needle for an insulin injection, the nurse would aspirate before depressing the plunger.

3. True or False: Before withdrawing insulin from the bottle or using a prefilled device, the nurse would shake the container vigorously to make sure the suspension is evenly distributed.

4. True or False: Prefilled pens and cartridges of insulin detemir (Levemir) would be stored at room temperature.

5. List three challenges to maintaining good control over blood glucose levels in pediatric patients.

   a. _____

   b. _____

   c. _____

6. Which nursing actions are important to take *after* giving a patient a noninsulin antidiabetic drug?

a. _____

b. _____

c. _____

NEXT-GENERATION NCLEX® EXAMINATION-STYLE CASE STUDY

Scenario: The nurse is caring for a 67-year-old patient with type 2 diabetes who was admitted with reports of abdominal pain and bloating. On assessment, the nurse notes the patient is hypotensive and the abdomen is distended. To assist in diagnosis, the provider has ordered a CT scan with contrast of the abdomen for the next day. The nurse reviews the electronic health record and notes the following:

Home Medications:
- Humalog insulin U-100 subcutaneously ac and hs as needed per sliding scale
- Metformin 850 mg orally twice daily with meals
- Aspirin 81 mg orally daily
- Carvedilol 25 mg orally daily

Highlight or underline the elements in the nursing assessment above that are of clinical significance.

PRACTICE QUIZ

____ 1. The nurse would instruct a pregnant patient that the last two trimesters of pregnancy would likely have which effect on the insulin needs of a patient with diabetes?
A. Increase during morning hours
B. Decrease at bedtime
C. Plateau at lunchtime
D. Overall increase

2. Which conditions can result from poorly controlled diabetes? *(Select all that apply.)*
____ A. Increased risk for infection
____ B. Increased sensitivity to touch
____ C. Elevated cholesterol levels
____ D. Kidney failure
____ E. Orthostatic hypotension

____ 3. A patient with diabetes who takes glucophage (Metformin) has postoperative orders to "resume all preoperative medications." What is the priority action for the nurse to take?
A. Follow the orders and resume all preoperative medications.
B. Hold all preoperative medications until verified with the pharmacy.
C. Contact the prescriber to obtain an order to hold the glucophage for 48 hours.
D. Hold oral preoperative medications until the patient has a bowel movement.

____ 4. A 68-year-old patient who is taking pioglitazone (Actos) will have which laboratory test done for follow-up?
A. Pulmonary function test (PFT)
B. Alanine transaminase (ALT)
C. Thyroid-stimulating hormone (TSH)
D. Complete blood count (CBC)

_____ 5. A patient has been prescribed exenatide (Byetta). Which patient statement indicates a correct understanding of the instruction given by the nurse?
   A. "I should keep this medication in the refrigerator, not the freezer."
   B. "Even if I miss breakfast, I should still take my exenatide."
   C. "This medication can cause weight gain, so I'll need to eat less."
   D. "This medication can cause me to feel hungrier between meals."

_____ 6. At 10 AM, a patient who was given an injection of Humulin R at 7:30 AM is anxious, has cool clammy skin, and noticeable hand tremors. What is the most likely explanation for these symptoms?
   A. The insulin is nearing the end of its duration of action.
   B. The insulin is having its peak effect, causing hypoglycemia.
   C. The patient likely ingested an excessive amount of carbohydrates.
   D. The patient has received an insufficient amount of insulin.

_____ 7. Which is the appropriate nursing action to ensure proper dosing before administering 50 units of Humulin N?
   A. Use a 5-mL syringe and administer 0.5 mL.
   B. Administer 50 units of insulin glargine.
   C. Ensure the vial contents are completely clear.
   D. Use a 50-unit or a 100-unit syringe.

_____ 8. Which method would the nurse use to teach a newly diagnosed patient with type 1 diabetes?
   A. Plan to provide one extended teaching session for the patient.
   B. Provide a variety of insulin syringes for the patient to examine.
   C. Ask the patient and the patient's caregiver to demonstrate back to you.
   D. Remind the patient that amputation could result if appropriate doses are not given.

_____ 9. The nurse is observing a colleague prepare to administer insulin by the subcutaneous route. The nurse would intervene and provide additional instruction under which circumstance?
   A. The colleague selects a 1-inch, 22-gauge needle for the injection.
   B. The colleague inserts the needle at a 45-degree angle for a thin patient.
   C. The colleague injects the insulin without first checking for a blood return.
   D. The colleague withdraws the needle rapidly after the injection is completed.

_____ 10. Which is the correct order of steps for combining two types of insulin into one syringe? (The dose to be given is 32 units of NPH and 8 units of regular insulin.)
   1. Draw up 8 units of air and inject into the regular vial.
   2. Ensure there is a total of 40 units in the syringe.
   3. Clean the tops of each vial with separate alcohol swabs.
   4. Draw up 32 units of NPH insulin into the syringe.
   5. Draw up 8 units of regular insulin into the syringe.
   6. Draw up 32 units of air and inject it into the NPH vial.

   A. 2, 3, 6, 1, 4, 5
   B. 3, 6, 1, 5, 4, 2
   C. 3, 1, 5, 6, 2, 4
   D. 2, 3, 4, 1, 5, 6

_____ 11. A patient is prescribed rosiglitazone (Avandia). The patient would be monitored for which adverse effect associated specifically with this drug?
   A. Lactic acidosis
   B. Difficulty digesting fatty meals
   C. Heart failure
   D. Kidney failure

_____ 12. The nurse has provided patient education about oral diabetic medications. Which patient statement indicates a need for additional teaching?
  A. "I will avoid drinking alcohol because I might not recognize hypoglycemia."
  B. "I will need to stay out of the sun while I am taking glipizide (Glucotrol)."
  C. "While I'm taking metformin (Glucophage), I can avoid the formation of lactic acid by drinking plenty of water."
  D. "I will take nateglinide (Starlix) twice daily with breakfast and dinner only."

Drug Therapy for Thyroid and Adrenal Gland Problems

LEARNING ACTIVITIES

Crossword Puzzle: Terminology Review

Complete the puzzle by identifying the correct words described in the clues below.

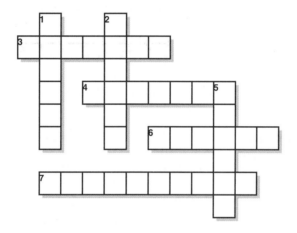

Across
3. An endocrine gland secretes a(n) _____.
4. The adrenal glands are located on top of the _____.
6. The target tissue of estrogen is the _____.
7. Thyroid hormones increase the rate of _____.

Down
1. The thick outermost layer of the adrenal gland is known as the _____.
2. Saltwater fish is a common dietary source of _____.
5. Cortisol (glucocorticoid) regulates the body's response to _____.

Fill in the Blank

1. Mitotane (Lysodren) works by directly inhibiting the _____ gland production of
   _____.

2. A medication to suppress adrenal hormone production is effective if the blood levels of
   _____ and _____ are reduced.

3. _____ is a hormone secreted by the adrenal cortex that regulates sodium and water balance.

4. _____ _____ _____ is a drug that mimics the effect of thyroid hormones to help regulate metabolism.

5. _____ are drugs similar to natural cortisol, a hormone secreted by the adrenal cortex that is essential for life.

6. A tissue or organ that is affected or controlled by a hormone is a(n) _____ _____.

7. The two thyroid hormones produced by the thyroid are _____ and _____.

8. _____ _____ and _____ _____ are common dietary sources of iodine.

9. _____ is the energy use of each cell, and the amount of work performed in the body.

10. Thyroid gland cells can divide, making the thyroid gland larger, causing a swelling in the neck called a(n) _____.

11. _____ is a severe type of hypothyroidism, which requires immediate medical attention.

12. Thyrotoxicosis is another term for _____ thyroid hormones.

Matching: Thyroid Disorders

Match the signs and symptoms with the correct thyroid disorder. (Answers may be used more than once.)

____ 13. Sleeping excessively

____ 14. Facial edema

____ 15. Feeling warm most of the time

____ 16. Rapid heart rate

____ 17. Weight gain

____ 18. Slowed speech

____ 19. Diarrhea

____ 20. Slow respiratory rate

A. Hypothyroidism
B. Hyperthyroidism

Identification: Thyroid Hormone Replacement Drugs

Indicate with an X whether the following precautions are Indicated or Contraindicated for patients who are taking thyroid hormone replacement drugs.

Precaution	Indicated	Contraindicated
21. Do not take these drugs during pregnancy.		
22. You can skip these drugs for up to a week if you are on vacation or do not feel well.		
23. Do not take a higher dose of the drug than what has been prescribed for you.		
24. Do not breastfeed an infant while taking these drugs.		
25. Go to the emergency department immediately if you have chest pain.		
26. If constipation occurs, stop the drug immediately.		
27. Take these drugs 3 hours before or 4 hours after taking a fiber supplement.		
28. These drugs enhance the activity of warfarin and increase the risk for excessive bleeding.		
29. These drugs decrease the activity of warfarin and increase the risk for blood clot formation.		
30. These drugs reduce the effectiveness of oral contraceptives.		

MEDICATION SAFETY PRACTICE

1. The nurse would teach a patient about the interaction between thyroid hormone replacement drugs and warfarin (Coumadin) because of the increased risk of _____.

2. Thyroid hormone replacement drugs would never be substituted for one another due to their variation in strengths, as well as the patient's _____.

3. A female patient who is of childbearing age and taking mifepristone is cautioned to use two forms of reliable contraception, because the drug can cause _____ _____.

4. A child who weighs 22 pounds is prescribed levothyroxine (Levothroid) 10 mcg/kg daily. How many mcg will the child receive each day? _____ mcg

5. A patient who is taking a thyroid hormone would be advised to take the drug at what time in regard to food or fiber supplement?

NEXT-GENERATION NCLEX® EXAMINATION-STYLE CASE STUDY

Scenario: A patient with Addison disease is being seen in the outpatient clinic for follow-up of medication therapy and to discuss the results of ordered laboratory studies. The patient has previously been prescribed a corticosteroid and fludrocortisone (Florinef). The nurse documents the following assessment:

"2+ edema noted to the lower extremities bilaterally. Patient reports some dyspnea with activity. Lung sounds clear."

The nurse notes that the patient's vital signs have changed since the last office visit 1 month prior.

Vital Signs

Date and Time	Temperature	Pulse	Respiration	Blood Pressure	Pulse Oximetry %O$_2$
May 10, 2023 1130	98.2° F oral	72 apical	18	126/78 mm Hg	98% room air
June 12, 2023 0800	98.2° F oral	96 apical	22	158/92 mm Hg	93% room air

Which condition(s) does the nurse suspect the patient is experiencing? **Select all that apply.**

____ A. Aldosterone deficiency
____ B. Hyperkalemia
____ C. Aldosterone excess
____ D. Hyponatremia
____ E. Cortisol excess

PRACTICE QUIZ

____ 1. Which statement by a patient who is taking thyroid replacement medication demonstrates a correct understanding of the therapy?
A. "As soon as my levels get back to normal, I can quit taking these pills."
B. "These pills will only serve to make me gain weight."
C. "I hope to feel better in general, and be more energetic during the day."
D. "I'll take this in the evening when I take my fiber supplement; that way I won't forget."

2. Which cardiac events may result from increased activity brought about by thyroid hormone replacement? *(Select all that apply.)*
____ A. Tamponade
____ B. Infarction
____ C. Heart block
____ D. Angina
____ E. Aortic stenosis
____ F. Heart failure

_____ 3. A patient who has Graves' disease has an endocrine disorder characterized by which action?
   A. The thyroid gland does not produce enough hormone.
   B. The body makes antibodies to thyroid-stimulating hormone, which bind to receptors.
   C. Antigens produced in the blood block hormone function.
   D. Slowed body metabolism causes decreased production of thyroid hormone.

_____ 4. Which statement best describes the mechanism of action of thyroid-suppressing drugs?
   A. Cells in the thyroid gland are killed by toxins and rendered unable to produce hormone.
   B. Thiamine is destroyed and cannot connect with iodine to make hormone.
   C. Hormones already formed and stored in the gland are depleted.
   D. The drug combines with the enzyme responsible for connecting iodide with tyrosine.

_____ 5. Which nursing action is crucial before administering thyroid replacement hormones?
   A. Administering the medication on the same schedule as at home
   B. Encouraging the patient to ask the pharmacist for a less-expensive brand
   C. Administering the medication with food to decrease stomach upset
   D. Dividing the prescribed medication into several doses throughout the day

_____ 6. An infant has been diagnosed with congenital absence of the thyroid gland. Which would the nurse emphasize during parent education?
   A. Most thyroid medications are prepared from nonallergenic animals.
   B. This medication is prescribed to promote mental and physical development.
   C. This medication will need to be taken only through adolescence.
   D. This medication eliminates the need for future monitoring of thyroid levels.

_____ 7. A patient asks the nurse, "How will I know when the thyroid replacement medication is working?" Which is the best response?
   A. "When your heart rate and blood pressure begin to decrease."
   B. "You probably will feel dramatically different within a week."
   C. "You will likely experience less constipation than previously."
   D. "You may begin to feel drowsier than you normally feel."

_____ 8. A patient with a history of a seizure disorder has had thyroid hormone recently prescribed. Which precaution would the nurse put in place?
   A. The patient should stop taking the thyroid hormone replacement.
   B. The patient will likely not experience any more seizures.
   C. The patient should take half of the prescribed antiseizure medications.
   D. The patient should be monitored for a higher risk of seizures.

_____ 9. The parent of a child who has had hypothyroidism since birth remarks, "He's gone through three shoe sizes in six months; he must be on a growth spurt!" What is an important aspect of care with thyroid replacement hormone treatment during rapid growth stages?
   A. The child will need an increase in the amount of replacement hormone.
   B. The child will be able to stop taking the thyroid replacement hormone.
   C. Growth spurts are common during childhood; no changes are needed.
   D. Further testing will likely now reveal the thyroid tissue has regrown.

10. The nurse is monitoring a patient with hyperthyroidism for symptoms of a thyroid crisis. Which symptoms are associated with this disorder? _(Select all that apply.)_
   _____ A. Hypothermia
   _____ B. Slow pulse
   _____ C. Hypertension
   _____ D. Fever
   _____ E. Lethargy

_____ 11. A patient who is pregnant has been diagnosed with hyperthyroidism. Which education will the nurse include in the patient's plan of care?
   A. The patient will be able to take additional doses of thyroid replacement hormone.
   B. Thyroid-suppressing medications are not generally prescribed during pregnancy.
   C. The patient will be able to take thyroid-suppressing drugs once she starts breastfeeding.
   D. The pregnant patient will be at a higher risk of infection, making surgical treatment unsafe.

_____ 12. Which is an assessment finding associated with adrenal gland hypofunction?
   A. Puffy, swollen facial features
   B. "Buffalo hump" noted on the back
   C. Overdeveloped muscles
   D. Darkening of the skin

_____ 13. Fludrocortisone (Florinef) is expected to cause which change?
   A. Lower the sodium level
   B. Reduce the potassium level
   C. Lower the blood pressure
   D. Lower the blood sugar

_____ 14. A patient taking an adrenal hormone-suppressing drug, mitotane (Lysodren) would have which change when the medication becomes effective?
   A. Normal growth pattern established
   B. Normal hair growth in place
   C. Reduced blood level of aldosterone
   D. Improved menstrual regularity

_____ 15. An older adult is taking thyroid suppressing medication. Which is an important consideration for this patient?
   A. Instruct the patient that blood clots are more likely to form.
   B. Recognize there is an increased risk for infection.
   C. The effects of warfarin are decreased.
   D. Adverse effects are less likely to be severe.

Drug Therapy for Seizures

LEARNING ACTIVITIES

Crossword Puzzle: Common Drug Names

Complete the puzzle by identifying the trade names of the antiseizure drugs that are described below in generic form.

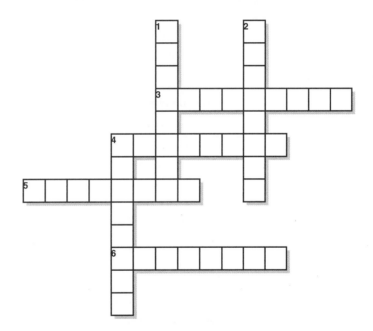

Across
3. gabapentin
4. valproic acid
5. primadone
6. carbamazepine

Down
1. clonazepam
2. ethosuximide
4. phenytoin

Matching: Terminology Review

Match the descriptions on the right with their correct terms on the left. (Answers may be used only once.)

_____ 1. Epilepsy
_____ 2. Myoclonic seizure
_____ 3. Seizure
_____ 4. Partial seizure
_____ 5. Aura
_____ 6. Status epilepticus
_____ 7. Absence seizure
_____ 8. Tonic-clonic seizure
_____ 9. Atonic seizure
_____ 10. Postictal phase
_____ 11. Generalized seizure

A. Blank stare, chewing movements, lasting less than 29 seconds
B. Sudden loss of muscle tone followed by confusion
C. Tingling, smell, or emotional changes occurring before a seizure
D. Brain disorder causing recurrent unprovoked seizures
E. Electrical discharges from both sides of the brain
F. Brief muscle jerk due to abnormal brain activity
G. Abnormal brain activity that starts in one part, may spread to the entire brain
H. Interval following a seizure featuring confusion, headache, and fatigue
I. Uncontrolled brain activity that may result in physical convulsion
J. Prolonged seizure or series of repeated seizures in a short interval
K. Stiffening or rigidity of arm and leg muscles with loss of consciousness

Fill in the Blank

List the medical term for each side effect of antiseizure medication below.

12. Loss of coordination, clumsiness _____

13. Double vision _____

14. Involuntary movements of the eyes _____

15. Excessive growth of gum tissue _____

16. Low platelet count _____

17. Low white blood cell count _____

Matching: Second-Line (Alternative) Drugs for Seizures

Match the descriptions on the right with the correct drugs on the left. (Answers may be used only once.)

_____ 18. clonazepam (Klonopin)
_____ 19. gabapentin (Neurontin)
_____ 20. phenobarbital (Luminal)
_____ 21. primidone (Mysoline)

A. Blocks or slows the spread of abnormal electrical impulses
B. Turns into phenobarbital in the body and blocks or slows the spread of abnormal electrical impulses
C. Stabilizes the membranes of neurons to decrease seizure activity
D. Action not well understood but most likely slows or stops transmission of abnormal electrical impulses

MEDICATION SAFETY PRACTICE

____ 1. Which action would the nurse take to reduce nausea and vomiting in a patient who is taking carbamazepine (Tegretol)?
   A. Give the medication early in the morning, before breakfast.
   B. Administer the drug at bedtime.
   C. Give the medication with food.
   D. Give the drug with an antacid.

2. Which are essential aspects of care for a patient who is experiencing a tonic-clonic seizure? *(Select all that apply.)*
   ____ A. Help the person to the floor.
   ____ B. Loosen clothing around the neck.
   ____ C. Place a padded tongue blade in the mouth.
   ____ D. Turn the person to the side.
   ____ E. Remove any sharp objects.
   ____ F. Administer an immediate oral dose of antiseizure medication.

____ 3. Which two antiseizure drugs may become habit-forming?
   A. Carbamazepine (Tegretol) and valproic acid (Depakote)
   B. Phenytoin (Dilantin) and ethosuximide (Zarontin)
   C. Primidone (Mysoline) and lamotrigine (Lamictal)
   D. Phenobarbital (Luminal) and clonazepam (Klonopin)

4. An older adult is more likely to experience which adverse effect from a first dose of phenytoin?

5. Although many drugs to treat seizures are considered category C or D, what are the risks to mother and fetus if a seizure occurs during pregnancy?

NEXT-GENERATION NCLEX® EXAMINATION-STYLE CASE STUDY

Scenario: A 22-year-old college student who has been recently diagnosed with focal seizures is in the medical clinic for a follow-up visit after being prescribed oxcarbazepine (Trileptal). The student reports dizziness, drowsiness, and headache.

Which instructions would the nurse give the patient regarding taking narrow-spectrum antiseizure drugs? **Select all that apply.**

____ A. "If you feel dizzy, skip a dose until the next day."
____ B. "These are common side effects; discuss them with your provider."
____ C. "Notify the clinic if you begin to experience bruising or unusual bleeding."
____ D. "Restrict your sodium intake while taking this drug."
____ E. "If you are taking birth control pills, you should use another form of contraception."
____ F. "Your provider may be able to prescribe alternative drugs that you can tolerate better."
____ G. "Remove all fall hazards in your home because this drug can cause clumsiness."
____ H. "Check your blood pressure regularly as this drug can cause hypertension."
____ I. "You will not need any lab tests with this medication."

PRACTICE QUIZ

____ 1. Which statement demonstrates a patient's understanding of therapy with valproic acid (Depakote)?
  A. "As soon as I stop having seizures, I will quit taking these pills."
  B. "If I miss a dose, I need to take it as soon as possible, but not if it would be doubling a regularly scheduled dose."
  C. "Since I have partial seizures, I only need to take part of one of these tablets."
  D. "If I notice slowed wound healing, I will call my doctor right away."

____ 2. The nurse would instruct a patient taking phenytoin to call the prescriber immediately if which condition develops?
  A. Excessive growth of hair in areas not normally hairy
  B. Overgrowth of gum tissue
  C. Difficulty coordinating movements
  D. Drowsiness

____ 3. The health care facility should plan to have which drug immediately available in the event a patient experiences status epilepticus?
  A. Diazepam (Valium)
  B. Phenytoin (Dilantin)
  C. Carbamazepine (Tegretol)
  D. Valproic acid (Depakote)

____ 4. Good oral hygiene is important for patients who are taking phenytoin (Dilantin) over long periods of time because of which side effect?
  A. Diplopia
  B. Nystagmus
  C. Hypertrichosis
  D. Gingival hyperplasia

____ 5. Which consideration is important for the nurse to remember for adolescents who are taking a first-line drug for generalized seizures?
  A. They often require decreased doses because of growth changes.
  B. They often require decreased doses because of hormonal changes.
  C. Sometimes they stop taking the medication to avoid gum changes.
  D. They often take extra doses to avoid noticeable skin changes.

____ 6. Which instruction is appropriate for the nurse to teach a pregnant patient who is taking a second-line drug for seizures?
  A. Dizziness is more common when taking lamotrigine (Lamictal).
  B. Reduce your folic acid intake when taking lamotrigine (Lamictal).
  C. Primidone (Mysoline) may cause clotting problems in newborns.
  D. Phenobarbital (Luminal) is associated with large-for-gestational-age fetuses.

____ 7. The nurse is obtaining a list of home medications for a patient who will be taking phenytoin (Dilantin) and an anticoagulant. Which interaction is possible between these two drugs?
  A. The effect of anticoagulants is decreased.
  B. Phenytoin tends to block the effect of anticoagulants.
  C. The dosage of phenytoin may need to be increased.
  D. The patient is at higher risk for bleeding.

____ 8. A patient experiences a seizure that lasts longer than 30 minutes. The nurse recognizes the patient experienced which type of seizure?
  A. Complex seizure
  B. Status epilepticus
  C. Partial seizure with secondary generalization
  D. Myoclonic seizure

____ 9. A patient taking an antiseizure drug should avoid which food item?
  A. Salted, cured bacon
  B. Grapefruit juice
  C. Eggs fried in butter
  D. High-fiber oatmeal

____ 10. A patient taking valproic acid (Depakote) has developed a nosebleed and bruises resulting from very minor injuries. This patient may be developing which adverse effect?
  A. Reduced red blood cells
  B. Increased white blood cells
  C. Increased red blood cells
  D. Reduced platelet count

____ 11. During the transfer process between facilities, a patient's prescription for phenytoin (Dilantin) was overlooked. Which complication could the patient experience?
A. The patient could develop seizures.
B. The patient's postictal stage is prolonged.
C. A more intense aura could occur.
D. Drug withdrawal symptoms are noted.

12. Which are possible consequences of exposure to phenytoin (Dilantin) during pregnancy? (*Select all that apply.*)
____ A. Drug withdrawal syndrome
____ B. Longer-than-normal fingernails
____ C. Increased risk for cleft palate
____ D. Growth deficiencies
____ E. Skull abnormalities

____ 13. A patient who takes carbamazepine (Tegretol) is discussing an upcoming vacation to a sunny beach location. Which special instruction is most crucial to provide for this patient?
A. Drink plenty of water to avoid dehydration.
B. Avoid overexertion with beachside sports.
C. Wear sunscreen to avoid skin sensitivity.
D. Increase the dosage to prevent stress-related seizures.

____ 14. A patient will be taking an antacid to deal with heartburn symptoms as well as phenytoin (Dilantin) to treat seizures. How can the nurse best help the patient schedule use of these medications?
A. Give the phenytoin 3 hours before taking the antacid.
B. To simplify the schedule, give the medications at the same time.
C. Give the antacid, then give the phenytoin 1 hour later.
D. Suggest to the patient that she decrease the antacid dose by half.

Drug Therapy for Alzheimer's and Parkinson's Diseases

chapter

24

LEARNING ACTIVITIES

Matching: Drug Names

Match each generic drug name on the right with its correct trade name on the left. (Answers may be used only once.)

____ 1. Namenda

____ 2. Aricept

____ 3. Exelon

____ 4. Reminyl

A. galantamine
B. rivastigmine
C. memantine
D. donepezil

Matching: Drug Categories

Match each category of drug on the right with the correct drug on the left. (Answers may be used more than once.)

____ 5. entacapone (Comtan)

____ 6. selegiline (Eldepryl)

____ 7. pramipexole (Mirapex)

____ 8. apomorphine (Apokyn)

____ 9. tolcapone (Tasmar)

____ 10. rasagiline (Azilect)

____ 11. benztropine (Cogentin)

____ 12. ropinirole (Requip)

____ 13. trihexyphenidyl (Artane)

____ 14. bromocriptine (Parlodel)

____ 15. carbidopa/levodopa (Sinemet)

A. Dopamine antagonist
B. COMT inhibitor
C. MAO-B inhibitor
D. Anticholinergic

Matching: Key Terms

Match the key term with its definition. (Answers may be used only once.)

____ 16. A progressive, incurable condition that destroys brain cells, gradually causing loss of intellectual abilities

____ 17. The loss of intellectual functions of sufficient severity to interfere with a person's daily functioning

____ 18. A unique type of cell found in the brain and body that is specialized to process and transmit information

____ 19. A chemical substance that transmits nerve impulses across a synapse

____ 20. A progressive disorder of the nervous system marked by muscle tremors, muscle rigidity, decreased mobility, stooped posture, slowed voluntary movements, and a masklike facial expression

A. Neuron
B. Alzheimer's disease
C. Dementia
D. Neurotransmitter
E. Parkinson's disease

Fill in the Blank

21. Cholinesterase/acetylcholinesterase inhibitors _____ the activity of the _____ acetylcholinesterase.

22. _____ _____ block cholinergic nerve impulses to help control muscle movements.

23. Dopaminergic/dopamine agonists increase the amount of _____ _____ in the brain.

24. Alzheimer's disease affects _____% of people over age 65, and as many as _____% of people over age 85.

25. Parkinson's disease most commonly begins between the ages of _____ and _____.

26. In Parkinson's disease, nerve cells degenerate in a part of the basal ganglia called the _____ _____.

MEDICATION SAFETY PRACTICE

____ 1. Before administering apomorphine (Apokyn), the nurse should obtain appropriate equipment to administer the medication by which route?
A. Oral
B. Intravenous
C. Intramuscular
D. Subcutaneous

____ 2. Which assessment would the nurse complete before administering oral medication to a patient with Alzheimer's disease due to the progressive effects of the disease?
A. Intake and output for the day
B. Vital signs
C. Ability to swallow
D. Daily weight

____ 3. Which instruction would the nurse provide to family and patients about administration of timed-release forms of medication?
   A. Always give with food.
   B. Do not give with grapefruit juice.
   C. Do not open or crush.
   D. Take with at least one full glass of water.

4. A patient with Parkinson's disease is prescribed ropinirole (Requip) 0.5 mg PO. The drug is available in scored tablets of 0.25 mg. How many tablets would the nurse give? _____ tablet(s)

5. A family member asks the nurse for assistance with "sorting out and organizing" medications for a patient who has Alzheimer's disease. Which medication is being given for which disorder?
   AcipHex _____   Aricept _____

NEXT-GENERATION NCLEX® EXAMINATION-STYLE CASE STUDY

Scenario: The home health nurse is caring for a patient with Alzheimer's disease who has recently been admitted. The patient has been prescribed the cholinesterase inhibitor donepezil (Aricept). The nurse is teaching the caregiver about this drug's effects.

Determine which responses from this Alzheimer's disease medication are a <u>COMMON SIDE EFFECT</u>, <u>ADVERSE EFFECT</u>, or sign of an <u>OVERDOSE</u> by placing an X in the appropriate column.

Response	Common Side Effect	Adverse Effect	Overdose
Nausea/vomiting			
Urinary retention			
GI bleeding			
Headaches			
Fatigue			
Drooling			
Anorexia			
Difficulty breathing			
Diarrhea			

PRACTICE QUIZ

____ 1. Which drug for Alzheimer's disease reduces the activity of the enzyme acetylcholinesterase that breaks down acetylcholine in the synapses of neurons?
   A. Memantine (Namenda)
   B. Galantamine (Reminyl)
   C. Entacapone (Comtan)
   D. Selegiline (Eldepryl)

2. A patient who is taking donepezil (Aricept) for Alzheimer's disease should be monitored for symptoms of which adverse effects? (*Select all that apply.*)
   ____ A. Seizures
   ____ B. Tachycardia
   ____ C. Atrial fibrillation
   ____ D. Muscle weakness
   ____ E. Weight gain

_____ 3. A nursing assistant in a long-term care facility reports that a patient with Alzheimer's disease choked several times during breakfast this morning. Which action is best to take before giving sustained-release galantamine (Razadyne) to this patient?
   A. Crush the medication and place it in applesauce or softened ice cream.
   B. Determine which food the patient enjoys and open the capsule onto it.
   C. Assess the patient's swallowing ability before giving the medication.
   D. Obtain the patient's height and weight to determine caloric needs.

_____ 4. Which statement by a family member indicates a correct understanding about the use of memantine (Namenda) for Alzheimer's disease?
   A. "I will administer this medication on an empty stomach."
   B. "This medication is also available in a skin patch."
   C. "This should improve the ability to perform complex tasks."
   D. "I will keep the medication stored in a safe location."

_____ 5. An older woman with Alzheimer's disease is very frail, weighing only 94 pounds. The nurse is reviewing the patient's medication record and notes that donepezil (Aricept) 10 mg PO at bedtime has been prescribed. Which is the best action to take?
   A. Administer the medication with food to avoid GI upset.
   B. Change the administration time to every morning.
   C. Ask the patient which food she would like the medication with.
   D. Consult with the prescriber about the drug dosage.

6. A patient is ordered pramipexole (Mirapex) to be given in three divided doses for a daily total of 4.5 mg. How many mg will each individual dose be?
   _____ mg

_____ 7. A patient who is taking entacapone (Comtan) reports feeling weak and achy recently. What question should the nurse ask the patient next?
   A. "What color is your urine?"
   B. "Have you lost more than 5 pounds in the last month?"
   C. "Do you have a fever?"
   D. "What color are the whites of your eyes?"
   E. "Have you had a bowel movement today?"

_____ 8. A patient who is taking ropinirole (Requip) to treat Parkinson's disease would be watched carefully for which potentially dangerous effect?
   A. Episodes of falling asleep suddenly
   B. Malignant melanoma
   C. Dyskinesia
   D. Rhinorrhea

_____ 9. A patient who is taking selegiline (Eldepryl) proudly announces he will be attending a college graduation party for his grandson. Which item must the patient avoid while taking this medication?
   A. Beer
   B. White wine
   C. Potato chips
   D. Pretzels

_____ 10. An older adult who is taking medication for Parkinson's disease would be cautioned to use extra care when walking because of which drug response?
   A. An increased risk for bradykinesia
   B. Rapid increase in blood pressure
   C. Confusion and hallucinations
   D. Rhinorrhea and excessive drooling

Drug Therapy for Psychiatric Problems

chapter

25

LEARNING ACTIVITIES

Crossword Puzzle: Common Drug Names

Complete the crossword puzzle by identifying the correct trade names for each drug described below in generic form.

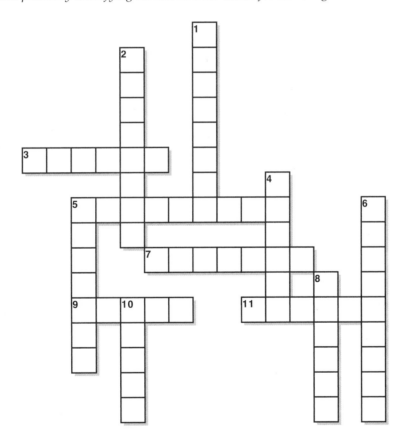

Across
3. fluoxetine
5. lithium carbonate
7. trazodone
9. paroxetine
11. thiothixene

Down
1. clonazepam
2. duloxetine
4. citalopram
5. escitalopram
6. risperidone
8. diazepam
10. alprazolam

Fill in the Blank

1. A selective serotonin reuptake inhibitor blocks the reuptake of _____, making it more available to act on _____ in the brain.

2. Tricyclic antidepressants act by blocking the reuptake of _____ and _____, making more of these substances available to act on receptors in the brain.

3. Other terms for an antipsychotic drug are _____ _____ and _____.

4. Another term for an antianxiety drug is _____.

5. Neuroleptic malignant syndrome is associated with _____ temperature, _____ pulse, _____, _____ respiratory rate, and _____ or _____ blood pressure.

Matching: Terminology Review

Match the descriptions on the right with their correct terms on the left. (Answers may be used only once.)

____ 6. Anxiety

____ 7. Bipolar disorder

____ 8. Depression

____ 9. Delusions

____ 10. Dysthymia

____ 11. Hallucinations

____ 12. Illusions

____ 13. Major depression

____ 14. Mania

____ 15. Obsessive-compulsive disorder

____ 16. Panic disorder

____ 17. Posttraumatic stress disorder

A. Alternating episodes of mania and depression
B. Fixed false beliefs or opinions that are resistant to reason
C. Feeling of dread about a perceived danger or threat
D. Incorrect mental representations of misinterpreted events
E. Feelings of sadness, despair, loss of energy, and difficulty coping
F. Sensory perceptions not actually present
G. Obsessive thoughts and compulsive actions
H. Persistently low moods; less severe than depression
I. Unexpected attacks of anxiety or terror lasting 15-30 minutes
J. Extremely elevated mood with mental and physical hyperactivity
K. Anxiety disorder caused by serious traumatic events
L. Persistent low mood and lack of pleasure in life with an increased risk of suicide

MEDICATION SAFETY PRACTICE

1. Patients taking venlafaxine, duloxetine, or bupropion are at risk for _____.

2. Patients on mirtazapine are at increased risk for infection because of _____.

3. Because of their abuse potential, _____ drugs are contraindicated for patients with a substance abuse disorder.

4. Patients taking quetiapine may experience an alteration in _____ _____ _____.

5. A patient has been prescribed chlorpromazine (Thorazine) 35 mg IM STAT. The medication is available in vials of 50 mg/2 mL. How many mL should be administered to the patient? _____ mL

NEXT-GENERATION NCLEX® EXAMINATION-STYLE CASE STUDY

Scenario: Joan is a 24-year-old woman with a diagnosis of paranoid schizophrenia and psychosis who is being seen in the outpatient mental health facility. Joan was previously prescribed fluphenazine (Prolixin) orally 5 mg twice daily. She has been taking it for 6 months with good resolution of psychotic symptoms, but she reports having headaches, constipation, and a recent urinary tract infection.

Determine which responses from fluphenazine are <u>COMMON SIDE EFFECTS</u>, <u>ADVERSE EFFECTS</u>, or <u>UNRELATED</u> to this medication by placing an X in the appropriate column.

Response	Common Side Effect	Adverse Effect	Unrelated
Weight gain			
Urinary tract infection			
Headache			
Tardive dyskinesia			
Neutropenia			
Constipation			

PRACTICE QUIZ

_____ 1. A patient who has been taking the benzodiazepine chlordiazepoxide (Librium) for anxiety reports after 2 weeks of therapy that she is feeling much calmer. This is a result of the enhanced inhibitory effects of which neurotransmitter?
A. Serotonin
B. Gamma-aminobutyric acid
C. Dopamine
D. Norepinephrine

_____ 2. A patient who was prescribed lorazepam (Ativan) for 2 months suddenly stopped taking it because she "felt so much better." Now she reports restlessness, weakness, and insomnia. The nurse would instruct her to call the prescriber and make an appointment immediately because of which risk associated with benzodiazepine withdrawal?
A. Sedation
B. Hypotension
C. Seizures
D. Stevens-Johnson syndrome

_____ 3. A patient who is in her second trimester of pregnancy is experiencing emotional difficulty at home and asks her health care provider for a prescription for lorazepam (Ativan) to help her cope. Why is this drug contraindicated for this patient?
A. It can cause birth defects.
B. The fetus can become dependent on the drug.
C. The risk of preeclampsia is increased.
D. It might make the patient miscarry.

_____ 4. A patient who has been taking sertraline (Zoloft) daily for 10 days reports that the medication has not helped with anxiety. What should the nurse tell the patient?
A. "This is a low dose and the prescriber will be contacted to request an increase."
B. "You should probably be taking a benzodiazepine for your condition."
C. "Another medication should be added to your regimen to get good results."
D. "You must give the drug more time because it is usually takes several weeks to be effective."

_____ 5. A patient has begun treatment with 25 mg of chlorpromazine (Thorazine) twice daily. You should instruct the patient to be sure to practice which precaution?
   A. Do not take the medication with grapefruit juice.
   B. Record daily weights to monitor for retained fluid.
   C. Change positions and get up slowly.
   D. Check fasting blood sugar daily.

   6. A patient has recently begun taking citalopram (Celexa) for symptoms of depression. You should monitor the patient for which common side effects? *(Select all that apply.)*
   _____ A. Insomnia
   _____ B. Anorexia
   _____ C. Dry mouth
   _____ D. Facial grimacing
   _____ E. Increased sweating

_____ 7. A group of individuals is participating in a support session to help with depression. Which patient statement would warrant the nurse to immediately notify the provider?
   A. "I still have feelings of extreme sadness every single day."
   B. "When will this medication start to work? I still cry a lot."
   C. "My mouth is so dry, I wish I had never started taking my medication."
   D. "If things don't improve, I'll have no reason to live anymore."

_____ 8. A patient who has taken chlorpromazine (Thorazine) has developed symptoms of muscle rigidity, elevated temperature, increased respiratory rate, and elevated pulse and blood pressure. In addition, the patient has become less responsive to verbal stimuli. Which adverse reaction has this patient developed?
   A. Tardive dyskinesia
   B. Neutropenia
   C. Neuroleptic malignant syndrome
   D. Myocarditis

_____ 9. Before giving clozapine (Clozaril) to a patient, the nurse assesses the patient's smoking history. What is the reason for this assessment?
   A. Hand tremors may cause self-injury while smoking.
   B. Smoking increases the risk of tardive dyskinesia.
   C. Smoking may decrease the effectiveness of clozapine.
   D. Smoking increases the risk of dementia.

_____ 10. Which statement made by a patient best indicates that the patient understands the correct use of olanzapine (Zyprexa)?
   A. "I won't worry if this drug causes my urine to turn pinkish-brown."
   B. "I won't take this drug with grapefruit juice to avoid excessive blood levels."
   C. "I can drink a glass of wine at night to help me relax and sleep better."
   D. "Suntanning is acceptable, as long as I do not use a tanning bed."

_____ 11. An older adult has been taking lithium and develops nausea and vomiting. Which intervention is most appropriate?
   A. Contact the prescriber for possible parenteral fluids.
   B. Remind the patient to restrict fluid intake.
   C. Hold the lithium until the nausea subsides.
   D. Instruct the patient about ways to restrict sodium intake.

Drug Therapy for Insomnia

LEARNING ACTIVITIES

Crossword Puzzle

Complete the puzzle by identifying the correct terms that are described.

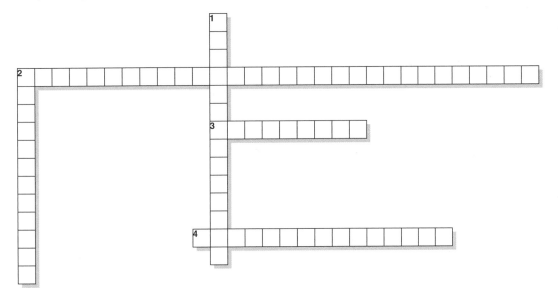

Across

2. A class of nonbenzodiazepine sedative-hypnotics that interacts with the same receptor site that benzodiazepine drugs do, turning on the receptors to induce sleep (three words)
3. Drugs that promote sleep by targeting signals in the brain to produce calm and ease agitation
4. A class of drugs that depress the CNS by binding to GABA receptors resulting in hypnotic and sedating effects; they are used mainly to control symptoms of anxiety or stress

Down

1. Drugs used to treat allergies and allergic reactions. Some, such as diphenhydramine (Allerdryl, Benadryl) and dimenhydrinate (Dramamine, Gravol), have sedating effects and are available over the counter
2. A class of drugs formed from barbituric acid that induces sedation and general depression over all CNS functions

Matching

Match each generic drug name on the right with its correct trade name on the left. (Answers may be used only once.)

_____ 1. Lunesta	A. zolpidem
_____ 2. Dalmane	B. zaleplon
_____ 3. ProSom	C. eszopiclone
_____ 4. Restoril	D. flurazepam
_____ 5. Ambien	E. estazolam
_____ 6. Sonata	F. temazepam
_____ 7. Doral	G. quazepam

Fill in the Blank

8. Benzodiazepines depress the CNS by binding to _____ _____.

9. _____ induce general depression over all CNS functions.

10. _____ and _____ function are inhibited by barbiturates.

11. Antihistamines produce _____ and _____ _____.

12. Drugs for insomnia are metabolized by the _____ and excreted by the _____.

MEDICATION SAFETY PRACTICE

1. A patient taking eszopiclone should be warned that serious adverse effects of this drug are _____ and _____ _____.

2. A patient with reduced liver function who is taking a drug to treat insomnia may have a(n) _____ drug level.

3. A patient has taken an overdose of a benzodiazepine. What is the reversal agent? _____ How is it administered? _____

4. A patient is to take 0.25 mg of triazolam (Halcion) at bedtime. The medication is available in 0.125-mg tablets. How many tablets should be administered? _____ tablets

5. Romazicon (Flumazenil) should not be given to a patient who has a(n) _____ _____.

NEXT-GENERATION NCLEX® EXAMINATION-STYLE CASE STUDY

Scenario: The nurse in the outpatient clinic is providing instructions to Mrs. Smith, a 68-year-old patient, who has been prescribed eszopiclone (Lunesta) for sleeplessness at night and irritability during the day. The patient lives alone with only her pets as companions.

Determine which nursing instructions related to taking eszopiclone are <u>CORRECT</u> and <u>INCORRECT</u> by placing an X in the appropriate column.

Instruction	Correct	Incorrect
"Take this medication when you have at least 7 hours of planned sleep time."		
"Keep a bright light on in your home in case you wake up."		
"Take this medication at least 2 hours before bedtime."		
"You may take another dose in 1 hour if the first dose isn't effective."		
"Have someone stay with you the first night you take the medication."		
"An herbal supplement like melatonin can be taken with this medication."		

PRACTICE QUIZ

_____ 1. Benzodiazepines are prescribed for short-term treatment for which reason?
A. They are excreted by the liver.
B. They are formed from barbituric acid.
C. They increase the seizure threshold.
D. They are habit-forming.

_____ 2. In addition to treatment for insomnia, barbiturates are used in management of which condition?
A. Chronic pain
B. Epilepsy
C. Depression
D. Psychosis

_____ 3. Which nursing intervention is most appropriate when administering a medication to treat insomnia?
A. Remind the patient to change positions slowly.
B. Administer the medication with a small glass of water.
C. Ask the patient to stay awake reading as long as possible.
D. Leave extra medication at the bedside in case the patient wants another dose.

_____ 4. A patient is taking a benzodiazepine receptor agonist for the first time at home. Which is the appropriate instruction for the nurse to give?
A. Turn off all the lights in the house, and sleep alone.
B. Take this medication about an hour before you go to bed.
C. Have another person stay with you the first time you take this.
D. Take this medication with an antihistamine, such as Benadryl.

_____ 5. A patient requests information about taking zolpidem during an overnight airplane flight that lasts 5-6 hours. Which information should the nurse provide?
A. This may cause a transient memory loss.
B. This is generally safe for most individuals.
C. Wine or alcohol can improve the drug's effect.
D. Stay awake during the flight, sleep upon arrival.

6. A child will be taking chloral hydrate (Aquachloral) prior to a CT scan that requires the child to be very still. The child weighs 44 pounds. How many mg should the child receive? _____ mg

____ 7. A patient has had an overdose of a benzo-diazepine. In addition to treatment with the reversal agent, the nurse will continue to monitor the patient for which adverse effect?
   A. Increased excitability
   B. Respiratory depression
   C. Elevated blood pressure
   D. Myocardial infarction

____ 8. Which considerations apply to an older adult who is taking a drug to treat insomnia?
   A. A higher dose is usually necessary.
   B. Safety precautions are necessary to prevent falls.
   C. Drug addiction is more likely to occur.
   D. Older adults are less sensitive to side effects.

____ 9. A mother who is breastfeeding an infant requests information on drugs to treat insomnia. Which information is most appropriate for the nurse to provide?
   A. These are usually safe to take while breastfeeding.
   B. The breastfed infant could be sedated by the medication.
   C. These drugs rarely enter into the breast milk.
   D. Take later at night to help you sleep better.

10. A patient will be taking flurazepam 30 mg this evening. The nurse will monitor the patient for which common side effects? *(Select all that apply.)*
   ____ A. Excess energy
   ____ B. Restlessness
   ____ C. Daytime drowsiness
   ____ D. Blurred vision
   ____ E. Confusion

Drug Therapy for Eye Problems

LEARNING ACTIVITIES

Matching: Terminology Review

Match the descriptions on the right with the correct terms on the left. (Answers will be used only once.)

_____ 1. Anterior chamber
_____ 2. Anterior segment
_____ 3. Aqueous humor
_____ 4. Conjunctiva
_____ 5. Glaucoma
_____ 6. Miosis
_____ 7. Mydriasis
_____ 8. Posterior chamber
_____ 9. Punctum
_____ 10. Posterior segment
_____ 11. Photoreceptors
_____ 12. Retina
_____ 13. Sclera

A. White outer layer of the eye
B. Clear membrane covering the front of the eye
C. Dilation of the pupil
D. Drains tears into the nasolacrimal sac
E. Back of the eye from the lens to the optic nerve
F. Increased intraocular pressure
G. Light-activated nerve endings
H. Clear fluid maintaining pressure and shape of the eye
I. Lining of the eye containing photoreceptors
J. Segment of the eye from the iris to the cornea
K. Constriction of the pupil
L. Part of the eye between the lens and the iris
M. Part of the eye between the lens and the cornea; contains chambers

Matching: Common Drug Names

Match the class of glaucoma drug on the right with the correct names on the left. (Answers may be used more than once.)

_____ 14. apraclonidine
_____ 15. carbachol
_____ 16. betaxolol
_____ 17. bimatoprost
_____ 18. acetazolamide
_____ 19. levobunolol
_____ 20. pilocarpine
_____ 21. latanoprost
_____ 22. methazolamide
_____ 23. carteolol
_____ 24. travoprost
_____ 25. timolol
_____ 26. dorzolamide
_____ 27. echothiophate
_____ 28. dipivefrin

A. Prostaglandin agonist
B. Beta-adrenergic blocking agent
C. Adrenergic agonist
D. Cholinergic
E. Carbonic anhydrase inhibitor

Matching: Drugs to Treat Glaucoma

Match the trade or brand name of each drug for glaucoma with its corresponding generic name. (Answers may be used only once.)

_____ 29. Diamox
_____ 30. Iopidine
_____ 31. Betoptic
_____ 32. Lumigan
_____ 33. Carboptic
_____ 34. Propine
_____ 35. Xalatan
_____ 36. Betagan
_____ 37. Ocusert
_____ 38. Timoptic
_____ 39. Travatan

A. timolol
B. latanoprost
C. betaxolol
D. apraclonidine
E. carbachol
F. dipivefrin
G. bimatoprost
H. levobunolol
I. pilocarpine
J. travoprost
K. acetazolamide

Fill in the Blank

40. An adrenergic agonist binds to the receptor sites in the eye that bind to naturally occurring _____ to reduce the amount of _____ humor produced.

41. _____ _____ _____ agents bind to adrenergic receptor sites and act as antagonists, preventing naturally occurring adrenalin from binding to the receptors.

42. _____ _____ _____ is a type of diuretic that lowers intraocular pressure by reducing production of aqueous humor.

43. A cholinergic agent increases the response that occurs when _____ binds to its receptor and activates it.

44. A prostaglandin agonist binds to prostaglandin receptor sites in the eye, causing eye blood vessels to _____, allowing blood vessels to _____, draining more _____ _____.

45. An intravitreal injection is a drug administration route in which the drug is injected into the _____ _____ of the eye.

46. Drugs that help lower intraocular pressure by decreasing episcleral venous pressure are _____ _____ _____.

MEDICATION SAFETY PRACTICE

_____ 1. Why is aseptic technique used to instill eyedrops?
   A. The eye is sterile.
   B. Eye medications are sterile.
   C. The eye is not well-protected by the immune system.
   D. Drug interactions may occur when multiple medications are administered.

_____ 2. Some drugs for the eye are also available as regular topical ointments. How are these formulations different?
  A. Neither preparation is sterile.
  B. The drug concentration in topical ointments is lower.
  C. Topical ointments are suspended in non–water-soluble carriers.
  D. The particles contained in the topical ointments are larger and should not be put in the eye.

3. The action performed to reduce systemic absorption of eye medication is known as
  _____ _____.

4. Prostaglandin agonists should only be used if the eye is _____.

5. Long-term use of beta blockers can increase the risk for _____.

6. In patients who have asthma or heart failure, _____ _____ drugs should be used with caution.

7. Patients who have taken MAO inhibitors within the last 2 weeks should not use _____ _____ eye medications.

8. If a patient is to be administered another eye medication after a carbonic anhydrase inhibitor, there should be an interval of _____ between instilling the two drugs.

NEXT-GENERATION NCLEX® EXAMINATION-STYLE CASE STUDY

Scenario: A 64-year-old woman is being seen at the primary care provider's office. The provider has diagnosed the patient with bacterial conjunctivitis secondary to contact lens use. The nurse is preparing to provide patient teaching regarding the proper use of prescribed eye medication.

Determine which nursing instruction is **INDICATED**, **CONTRAINDICATED**, or **NONESSENTIAL** for the administration of eye medications by placing an X in the appropriate column.

Instruction	Indicated	Contraindicated	Nonessential
"Wash your hands before administering eye drugs."			
"Remove contact lenses before applying the medication."			
"Wash the eye with warm tap water before administration."			
"When two types of eyedrops are prescribed, mix them together and then apply."			
"Before applying ointment, first squeeze out some of the ointment onto a tissue and discard it."			
"Try to center the drop right over the pupil."			
"After applying eyedrops, apply pressure over the inside corner of the eye."			
"After applying eye ointment, tape the eyelids closed for 1 hour."			
"Wear an eyepatch when sleeping."			

PRACTICE QUIZ

_____ 1. When an eye appears "bloodshot," the vessels that are visible are in what part of the eye?
A. Sclera
B. Pupil
C. Aqueous humor
D. Conjunctiva

_____ 2. An older adult patient with diabetes who is taking beta blockers for glaucoma must be instructed to perform what assessment?
A. Daily weight
B. Intake and output
C. Blood glucose level
D. Urine ketones

_____ 3. Which is most important to assess before administering a prostaglandin agent to a patient?
A. Corneal color changes
B. Excessive eyelash growth
C. Presence of cataracts
D. Whether the eye surface is intact

_____ 4. What teaching point must be included for a patient who is taking cholinergic drugs for treatment of glaucoma?
A. Wear sunglasses when reading fine print indoors.
B. Limit your fluid intake to less than 2000 mL per day.
C. Apply punctal pressure for 10 minutes to avoid systemic effects.
D. Use caution in dim lighting to prevent falls and injury.

_____ 5. A patient had an allergic reaction to a sulfa antibiotic 1 year ago. This indicates that the patient may have sensitivities to which eye medication?
A. Carbonic anhydrase inhibitors
B. Cholinergics
C. Prostaglandin agonists
D. Adrenergic blockers

_____ 6. The rationale for pressing on the inner canthus after instilling eyedrops is to avoid what event?
A. Overdosage
B. Contamination
C. Systemic side effects
D. Increased intraocular pressure

_____ 7. A middle-aged patient with glaucoma is not following the prescribed regimen for instilling eyedrops. He says he can see just fine and his eyes do not hurt. What factors regarding glaucoma should be reviewed with him?
A. Vision damage from glaucoma occurs painlessly.
B. When the pain from glaucoma returns, resume eyedrop use.
C. When difficulty seeing occurs, resume eyedrop use.
D. Your central vision would be affected first with glaucoma.

_____ 8. A patient has been taught how to apply bimatoprost (Lumigan) eyedrops to treat glaucoma in the affected right eye. Which patient action indicates the need for further teaching?
A. The patient administers the correct number of drops to both eyes.
B. The drops are applied to the pocket of the lower lid of the eye.
C. The patient avoids touching the eye with the tip of the bottle.
D. The patient wipes away excess drops from the face with a tissue.

_____ 9. Which assessment finding is most likely associated with use of travoprost (Travatan) for several months?
A. Cloudiness of the lens
B. Bulging of the eye tissues
C. Darkening of the iris
D. Unequal pupil size

_____ 10. A patient has been taking timolol (Timoptic) eyedrops for several months and recently experienced a decreased pulse and worsening of asthma symptoms. What is the most likely explanation for this?
A. The patient took the timolol orally, instead of administering to the eyes.
B. The patient used the drops in both eyes instead of just one.
C. The patient abruptly stopped using the prescribed eyedrops.
D. The patient did not apply pressure to the punctum after administration.

Drug Therapy for Male Reproductive Problems

chapter
28

LEARNING ACTIVITIES

Matching

Match the descriptions on the left with the correct terms on the right. (Answers may be used only once, and not all options may be used.)

_____ 1. Enlargement of the prostate gland is called benign prostatic _____ (BPH).
_____ 2. A reduced _____ of the urine stream is also a symptom of BPH.
_____ 3. The amount of circulating testosterone _____ with aging
_____ 4. A patient with BPH should be seen by the health care provider to rule out _____ cancer.
_____ 5. The prostate gland surrounds the upper part of the _____.
_____ 6. A symptom of BPH is increased _____ of urination.
_____ 7. Male hormone produced in the testes is _____.

A. Urethra
B. Prostate
C. Force
D. Frequency
E. Decreases
F. Hyperplasia
G. Penis
H. Bladder
I. Testosterone
J. Increases
K. Hypertrophy

Identification: Drug Categories

Place an 'X' in the column to the right of each drug that corresponds with the correct drug category.

Drug	DHT Inhibitors	Selective Alpha-1 Blockers	Testosterone Drugs	Erectile Dysfunction Drugs
8. testosterone gel (AndroGel)				
9. dutasteride (Avodart)				
10. doxazosin (Cardura)				
11. tamsulosin (Flomax)				
12. testosterone patch (Androderm)				
13. terazosin (Hytrin)				
14. finasteride (Proscar)				
15. vardenafil (Levitra)				

MEDICATION SAFETY PRACTICE

____ 1. The nurse is working with a patient who is taking dutasteride (Avodart) 5 mg daily. The patient's granddaughter, who is in the second trimester of pregnancy, says she wants to cut the tablets in half so the patient can swallow them easily. What should be the nurse's response?
A. "These can easily be broken in half. Just make sure to give him both halves."
B. "You should not handle these tablets, especially when they are cut in half."
C. "You need to move out of your grandfather's house while he is taking this drug."
D. "If cutting them in half doesn't work, crush them and put them in applesauce."

2. A patient with impaired liver function should not take finasteride (Proscar) for which reason?

3. A patient is taking finasteride (Proscar) and states he is still sexually active with his wife, who is now pregnant. What special teaching is necessary?

4. A patient who is taking tamsulosin (Flomax) is having cataract eye surgery in a week. What problem can occur during this surgery?

5. Testosterone is pregnancy category _____.

NEXT-GENERATION NCLEX® EXAMINATION-STYLE CASE STUDY

Scenario: Joseph Smith, a 65-year-old retired teacher, is being seen in the urology clinic for follow-up after a diagnosis of benign prostatic hyperplasia (BPH). The nurse is preparing to teach Mr. Smith about the medications that the provider has prescribed to him.

Complete the following teaching points the nurse should include by choosing from the list of options below.

"Your provider has prescribed finasteride, a DHT inhibitor. DHT inhibitors should be used with caution with the herbal supplements _____1_____ and _____1_____. A DHT inhibitor may cause a slowing of ____2____ from the scalp. Your provider has also prescribed tamsulosin, a selective alpha blocker drug. This medication relaxes _____3_____ in the bladder neck. Tamsulosin may cause an allergic reaction in patients who are allergic to _____4_____."

Options for 1	Options for 2	Options for 3	Options for 4
garlic	hair thickness	smooth muscle	finasteride
saw palmetto	hair loss	the urethra	tetracycline
echinacea	flaking	the prostate gland	opioids
St. John's wort	redness	urine	sulfa drugs
soy isoflavones		calculi	penicillin

PRACTICE QUIZ

_____ 1.   A patient has been educated about taking his first dose of doxazosin (Cardura). What patient statement indicates the need for further instruction?
   A.   "I'll take this medication at night, right before I go to bed."
   B.   "I'll take this medication before I drive to work in the morning."
   C.   "If I get dehydrated, I'm more likely to get dizzy when I stand up."
   D.   "My son is staying with me the first night I take it, in case I need to get up."

_____ 2.   An older male patient taking a drug for benign prostatic hyperplasia needs to visit his health care provider annually for which reason?
   A.   Pharmacies will not renew the prescription without an annual refill order.
   B.   Older adults are more likely to develop heart failure and hypertension.
   C.   Prostate cancer is more likely to occur in males during the aging process.
   D.   The drug tends to be less effective with aging and the dose needs to be increased.

   3.   A patient is to receive an IM injection of testosterone cypionate 150 mg IM. The vial is labeled 200 mg/mL. What is the amount to be given? _____ mL

_____ 4.   Which assessment finding is a common side effect of treatment with testosterone?
   A.   Dry, scaly skin
   B.   Enlarged testicles
   C.   Pitting ankle edema
   D.   Breast enlargement

_____ 5.   Which patient should _not_ receive treatment with testosterone?
   A.   A patient with a history of breast cancer
   B.   A patient with a decreased interest in sex
   C.   A patient with decreased bone density
   D.   A patient with depression and irritability

_____ 6.   To avoid virilization effects in women exposed to testosterone gel or patches, which precaution should be in place?
   A.   The clothing and linen used by the man should be hand-washed, not machine-laundered.
   B.   It is safe for the woman to apply the testosterone gel, as long as she washes her hands afterwards.
   C.   Avoid touching the skin, clothing, or linen that has been in contact with the testosterone gel.
   D.   The patch can be placed or removed by a female, as long as she washes her hands afterwards.

_____ 7.   Which is a physiologic risk factor for erectile dysfunction?
   A.   Depression
   B.   Diabetes
   C.   Anxiety
   D.   Stress

_____ 8.   Phosphodiestrase-5 inhibitor drugs help with erectile dysfunction in which manner?
   A.   Relax smooth muscles and allow the penis to fill with blood
   B.   Contract voluntary muscles to improve blood flow to the penis
   C.   Allow penile erection to occur in the absence of sexual stimulation
   D.   About 10 minutes after taking the drug, an erection is likely to occur

_____ 9.   A patient mentions having a headache after using sildenafil (Viagra). The patient can be advised to use the recommended dose of which medication to treat these symptoms?
   A.   Acetaminophen (Tylenol)
   B.   Hydrocodone (Norco)
   C.   Doxazosin (Cardura)
   D.   Sublingual nitroglycerine

10. A patient is taking a drug to treat BPH symptoms. Which indicates the medication is effective? *(Select all that apply.)*
    ____ A. Less difficulty starting the urine stream
    ____ B. A feeling of bladder fullness
    ____ C. A reduction in sexual libido
    ____ D. Needing to urinate less frequently at night
    ____ E. Improved overall body strength

____ 11. Which side effect of dutasteride (Avodart) has future reproductive implications?
    A. Decreased fertility
    B. Births of multiples
    C. Increased libido
    D. Increased seminal fluid

Drug Therapy for Female Reproductive Problems

LEARNING ACTIVITIES

Crossword Puzzle: Terminology Review

Complete the puzzle by identifying the key terms that are described.

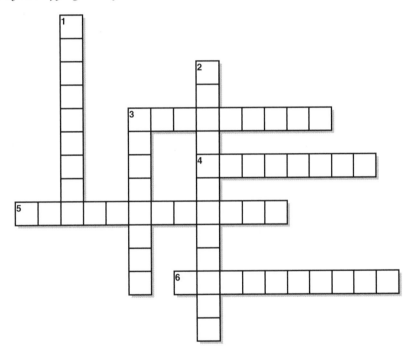

Across
3. The cessation of menstrual periods and ovulation
4. The main female sex hormone secreted by the ovaries
5. The periodic shedding of the uterine lining
6. The ovum is fertilized by a sperm

Down
1. The release of a mature ovum
2. The female hormone that supports pregnancy by maintaining the thickened uterine lining
3. The term for the beginning of the years of menstruation

Matching

Match the definition on the left with the correct term on the right. (Answers may be used only once.)

_____ 1.   Shedding of the uterine lining

_____ 2.   Beginning of the years of menstruation during adolescence

_____ 3.   Interest in sexual activity

_____ 4.   Cessation of menstrual periods and ovulation

_____ 5.   Glandular cells in the ovary shrink and become nonfunctional

_____ 6.   Transition between having regular menstrual cycles to time
           when menstrual periods have stopped for a full year

_____ 7.   Blood vessels dilating, causing uncomfortable symptoms

_____ 8.   Mature ovum is fertilized by a sperm

A. Menarche
B. Hot flashes
C. Menstruation
D. Perimenopause
E. Menopause
F. Libido
G. Pregnancy
H. Involution

Fill in the Blank

9.   _____ is the main female hormone secreted by the ovaries and adrenal glands.

10. Follicle-stimulating hormone causes the ovary to secrete estrogen, allowing one ovum in the ovary to
     _____ _____ each month.

11. _____ _____ causes secretion of progesterone by the ovary and al-
     lows the release of a mature ovum.

12. Progesterone supports pregnancy by maintaining the thickened _____
     _____.

13. Dropping levels of estrogen and progesterone allow the lining of the uterus to stop growing, and to be
     shed as _____.

14. If conception occurs, the fertilized ovum implants into the uterine lining within ____ to ____ days.

15. When the glandular cells of the ovary shrink, they no longer produce normal levels of
     _____.

MEDICATION SAFETY PRACTICE

1.   Estrogen-based hormone replacement therapy is not recommended for long-term therapy due to which
     concern?

2.   A patient who is considering use of estrogen-based hormone replacement therapy smokes. What advice
     would the nurse give, and why?

3.   In women who still have a uterus and are taking perimenopausal HRT, the uterine lining can thicken,
     causing which problem?

4. Which type of cancers are hormone-sensitive and whose growth can be increased by perimenopausal HRT?

5. Perimenopausal HRT can increase the risk for which gastrointestinal disorders?

NEXT-GENERATION NCLEX® EXAMINATION-STYLE CASE STUDY

Scenario: The nurse is interviewing a 23-year-old sexually active female who has come to the provider's office seeking birth control. The patient smokes a half-pack of cigarettes per day. The provider prescribes oral contraceptive medication.

Which statements made by the patient indicate a correct understanding of taking oral contraceptive medication? **Select all that apply.**

____ A. "I should take these pills on an empty stomach."
____ B. "I can take this medication at any time each day."
____ C. "If I miss one dose in a cycle, the medication should still be effective."
____ D. "I'll need to follow up with my provider if I see yellowing of my eyes or darkening of my urine."
____ E. "I can continue taking this medication if I become pregnant."
____ F. "I would still need my partner to use a condom to prevent HIV."
____ G. "I do not need to take more than one dose a day."
____ H. "I should report pain or swelling of my leg to my provider immediately."

PRACTICE QUIZ

____ 1. A woman has been provided instructions on use of oral contraceptives. Which patient statement indicates the need for further instructions?
A. "If I miss one dose, I should throw all the pills away, and start a new pack in a month."
B. "I should plan on using a barrier method, such as a condom for the first month on the pill."
C. "If I miss one dose within a cycle, the drug should still be effective to prevent pregnancy."
D. "If I miss two doses, I should use another type of contraceptive while continuing the pill."

____ 2. A patient undergoing menopause asks, "How will I know if the hormone replacement therapy is working?" Which is the nurse's best response?
A. "Your menstrual cycles will eventually become more regular."
B. "Your symptoms of hot flashes and night sweats will lessen."
C. "Your menstrual cycles will become less painful and less heavy."
D. "Your symptoms of fluid retention and weight gain will improve."

____ 3. A patient has recently begun taking HRT. During subsequent visits, the patient would be assessed for which common side effect of HRT?
A. Weight loss
B. Facial hair growth
C. Fluid retention
D. Scalp hair loss

____ 4. A patient is to be monitored for liver dysfunction after beginning HRT. Which assessment findings are associated with liver dysfunction?
   A. Pale, waxy skin
   B. Oral cyanosis
   C. Yellow tinge to the skin
   D. Ruddy face

____ 5. A young adult requests information about various forms of contraception. Which form of contraception is most reliable?
   A. Oral contraceptive pills
   B. Implanted contraceptives
   C. Condoms and spermicides
   D. Complete abstinence

____ 6. Oral contraceptives are effective for which reason?
   A. The uterus lining sheds more often.
   B. Ovulation does not occur.
   C. Menstrual cycles are more frequent.
   D. The uterine lining thickens.

____ 7. A patient mentions she has heard of the "mini-pill" and requests information about this. Which information should the nurse provide?
   A. It raises the blood level of progesterone.
   B. It decreases the blood level of estrogen.
   C. It is smaller and easier to swallow.
   D. It is to be taken only once a month.

____ 8. A patient is having her annual physical exam and renewal of her prescription of drospirenone/estradiol (Angelique). What is the most likely reason she is scheduled for a blood test today?
   A. To determine if she is using the medication as prescribed.
   B. To determine whether her potassium level is elevated.
   C. To determine if her estrogen levels are still sufficient.
   D. To determine if she has bone marrow cancer.

____ 9. A patient has been provided information about oral contraceptives. Which patient statement indicates the need for further education?
   A. "I'll need to take this medication at the same time every day."
   B. "I'll make sure to keep getting screened for cervical cancer."
   C. "I'm glad I won't be exposed to any sexually transmitted diseases."
   D. "I'll need to discuss any new medications with the provider."

____ 10. Children should not take either hormone replacement drugs or hormonal contraception before puberty for which reason?
   A. Its use has been associated with kidney disease.
   B. Children are more likely to develop breast cancer.
   C. Deep vein thrombosis is more likely to occur.
   D. This may cause growth of the long bones to stop.

____ 11. A mother who is breastfeeding her infant should not use hormonal contraception for which reason?
   A. It is likely to interfere with lactation.
   B. Breastfeeding is a natural contraceptive.
   C. It changes the contour of the breasts.
   D. It changes the breast milk nutrients.

Notes

Notes